Contemporary Endocrinology

Contemporary Endocrinology offers an array of titles covering clinical as well as bench research topics of interest to practicing endocrinologists and researchers. Topics include obesity management, androgen excess disorders, stem cells in endocrinology, evidence-based endocrinology, diabetes, genomics and endocrinology, as well as others. Series Editor Leonid Poretsky, MD, is Chief of the Division of Endocrinology and Associate Chairman for Research at Lenox Hill Hospital, and Professor of Medicine at Hofstra North Shore-LIJ School of Medicine.

Sarah Fishman
Editor

Advances in Diabetes Technology

Springer

Editor
Sarah Fishman
Premier Endocrine
New York, NY, USA

ISSN 2523-3785 ISSN 2523-3793 (electronic)
Contemporary Endocrinology
ISBN 978-3-031-75351-0 ISBN 978-3-031-75352-7 (eBook)
https://doi.org/10.1007/978-3-031-75352-7

This Springer imprint is published by the registered company Springer Nature Switzerland AG
The registered company address is: Gewerbestrasse 11, 6330 Cham, Switzerland

Foreword

As the diabetes epidemic continues to advance both in the United States and worldwide, the specific causes of most forms of diabetes mellitus as well as the cure continue to elude us. Some good news regarding diabetes mellitus, however, should not be ignored: with improved therapies the rates of both cardiovascular and microvascular complications are beginning to decline [1].

With some important exceptions [2], glycemic control continues to be a very important contributor to a reduction in complication rates for both type 1 and type 2 diabetes mellitus [3–6]. In addition, the advent of revolutionary medical therapies (such as SGLT-2 inhibitors and GLP1/GIP receptor agonists) and advances in diabetes mellitus technology for both glucose monitoring and the modes of insulin delivery (as well as their combinations) have been progressing at a breakneck speed.

The current volume of *Contemporary Endocrinology*, masterfully edited by Sarah Fishman, MD, PhD, provides a timely summary of the latter group of these advancements. It covers both the historical perspectives and the current state of diabetes technology in all of its aspects. The authors of all chapters are not only established investigators, but also prominent clinical practitioners, making this book extremely useful as a practical guide for a busy clinician.

The editor and the authors deserve congratulations on this important accomplishment.

New York, NY, USA Leonid Poretsky

References

1. Gregg EW, Li Y, Wang J, Rios Burrows N, Ali MK, Rolka D, Williams DE, Geiss L. Changes in diabetes-related complications in the United States, 1990–2010. N Engl J Med. 2014;370:1514–23. https://doi.org/10.1056/NEJMoa1310799.
2. Action to Control Cardiovascular Risk in Diabetes Study Group, Gerstein HC, Miller ME, Byington RP, Goff DC Jr, Bigger JT, Buse JB, Cushman WC, Genuth S, Ismail-Beigi F, Grimm RH Jr, Probstfield JL, Simons-Morton DG, Friedewald WT. Effects of intensive glucose

lowering in type 2 diabetes. N Engl J Med. 2008;358(24):2545–59. https://doi.org/10.1056/NEJMoa0802743. Epub 2008 Jun 6. PMID: 18539917; PMCID: PMC4551392.
3. Diabetes Control and Complications Trial Research Group, Nathan DM, Genuth S, Lachin J, Cleary P, Crofford O, Davis M, Rand L, Siebert C. The effect of intensive treatment of diabetes on the development and progression of long-term complications in insulin-dependent diabetes mellitus. N Engl J Med. 1993;329(14):977–86. https://doi.org/10.1056/NEJM199309303291401. PMID: 8366922.
4. Nathan DM, Cleary PA, Backlund JY, Genuth SM, Lachin JM, Orchard TJ, Raskin P, Zinman B, Diabetes Control and Complications Trial/Epidemiology of Diabetes Interventions and Complications (DCCT/EDIC) Study Research Group. Intensive diabetes treatment and cardiovascular disease in patients with type 1 diabetes. N Engl J Med. 2005;353(25):2643–53. https://doi.org/10.1056/NEJMoa052187. PMID: 16371630; PMCID: PMC2637991.
5. King P, Peacock I, Donnelly R. The UK prospective diabetes study (UKPDS): clinical and therapeutic implications for type 2 diabetes. Br J Clin Pharmacol. 1999;48(5):643–8. https://doi.org/10.1046/j.1365-2125.1999.00092.x. PMID: 10594464; PMCID: PMC2014359.
6. Holman RR, Paul SK, Bethel MA, Matthews DR, Neil HA. 10-year follow-up of intensive glucose control in type 2 diabetes. N Engl J Med. 2008;359(15):1577–89. https://doi.org/10.1056/NEJMoa0806470. Epub 2008 Sep 10. PMID: 18784090.

Contents

Chapter 1
Introduction

Jeffrey Unger

At the age of 15, Roy was diagnosed as having type 1 diabetes. The year was 1965 when the mortality rate for patients under the age of 30 was 10% and over 40% for patients older than age 60 [1]. The global prevalence of diabetes in 1965 was estimated to be 30 million (1% of the global population). Today over 579 million people worldwide are living with diabetes representing 7% of the global population [1].

Roy was advised by his physician to "enjoy your next 5 years of life, because you will not live beyond the age of 20." Roy, for the most part, remained adherent to his insulin regimen, taking his pork or beef insulin 70 units in the AM using reusable glass syringes and needles which were boiled and sanitized every morning prior to use. The needles were reused until the injections in his legs became unbearably painful that he was forced to replace them. Roy was able to participate in sporting events, hang out with friends and enjoy life with the full expectation that he would be dead by the age of 20. Thankfully, Roy continues to thrive today at the tender age of 75. In 1997, he was placed on his first insulin pump. He continued to do multiple finger sticks each day and learned to adjust the dose of his prandial insulin based on his predicted food intake, activity level, and pre-prandial glucose levels.

In 2006 while driving on an LA freeway, Roy (age 56) collided with five different cars before coming to rest on the shoulder of the road. A CHP officer noted that Roy appeared dazed, confused, and disoriented while sitting alone in the front seat of his car. "Sir, are you OK? Do you know what just happened?" Roy responded, "No sir, why are you asking me these questions?" An ambulance arrived on scene and transported Roy to the local emergency room where his blood glucose level was 39 mg/dL. Roy's driving privileges were immediately suspended and he was told that he would have to go to court where a judge would determine if his driving privileges would be terminated.

J. Unger (✉)
Unger Primary Care Concierge Medical Group, Rancho Cucamonga, CA, USA
e-mail: jungermd@aol.comH

S. Fishman (ed.), *Advances in Diabetes Technology*, Contemporary Endocrinology, https://doi.org/10.1007/978-3-031-75352-7_1

Following the suspension of his license Roy began to exhibit signs of clinical depression. Rather than initiating antidepressant medications or offering behavioral intervention, Roy was provided with a newly released Dexcom 4 continuous glucose monitoring device. The Dexcom 4 transmitted interstitial glucose values every 5 min to a "reader" which alarmed when glucose values trended towards hypoglycemia. After wearing the device for a month, Roy downloaded the data from each 24 h period and presented his "portfolio" to the traffic court magistrate. The judge called a short recess so that she could review the sensor data in more detail. She later admitted that she had never seen this kind of data in her 30 years on the bench.

When Court resumed, her Honor said, "Roy, this is so impressive. I have to tell you, that when you wear your sensor you are the safest driver on the road. I am not going to restrict your right to operate a motor vehicle in any way. However, I am ordering you to always where this amazing device whenever you drive. Oh, and by the way, I think I'm going to ask my Mother's physician to get her one as well!"

Prior to the discovery of insulin in 1922 the mortality rates for patients with diabetes exceeded 824 per 1000 patient years. Fortunately, the rates declined significantly to fewer than 1% per 1000 patient years in 1961 as patients were placed on insulin therapy [2]. A CDC and prevention analysis of diabetes-related mortality prior to age 20 years showed a decrease of 61% (2.7 deaths per million per year in 1968–1969 vs 1.0 deaths per million per year in 2008–2009). Although patients began to live longer with diabetes, they faced a high risk of developing long-term complications such as DKA, hypoglycemia, cardiovascular disease, infectious diseases, and renal impairment [3].

In the 1970s, Roy was advised by his physicians to "keep your blood sugar as low as possible, because high glucose levels will increase your risk of developing complications." A paradigm shift has now occurred which portends an increased risk of hospitalizations and mortality rates in patients experiencing severe hypoglycemia. Between 1999 and 2011 Black patients experienced higher rates of hypoglycemia and hyperglycemia compared with white patients. Additionally, adults age 75 and older had higher rates of hospital admissions related to hypoglycemia [4]. Interstitial glucose monitoring technology can provide users with real-time and trending glucose values every minute of every day. These devices can alarm and warn patients of impending hypoglycemia events allowing the user to act quickly and effectively to reverse rapid declines in glucose levels. In contrast, patients who use self-blood glucose monitoring will not be able to determine a hypoglycemic event unless they are fortunate enough to test when hypoglycemic.

The introduction of continuous subcutaneous insulin infusion pumps in 1974 allowed patients with diabetes to experience a more physiologic insulin delivery modality. The prototype of an insulin pump designed by Dr. Arnold Kadish in 1963 was worn as a back pack [5]. In 1983, MiniMed introduced their first insulin pump, MiniMed 502. This system soon underwent significant improvements in size and programmability and thus represented a major technologic breakthrough in the evolution of insulin pumps. The pump, which featured metal bent needle infusion catheters, allowed patients to minimize their dependency on multiple daily injections by providing a programed basal rate infusion of rapid acting insulin coupled with the patient's ability to bolus mealtime insulin through the device. The new generation external pumps, released in the 1990s, are comparatively small, compact, handy, and effective. These "smart pumps" have features such as built-in bolus calculators, personal computer interfaces, and occlusion alert alarms. Table 1.1 lists the currently approved insulin pumps available in the USA.

Table 1.1 Insulin pump devices available in the US market

Insulin pump name	Unique features
Medtronic 670 G	• Hybrid closed loop featuring SmartGuard technology allowing users to choose between increasing levels of automation which best fit the needs of their diabetes self-management • SmartGuard technology can halt insulin delivery for up to 2 h for treatment emergent impending hypoglycemia • Works with CareLink personal software to incorporate CGM with insulin delivery • Approved for use by adults and children over the age of 14 with type 1 diabetes
Aviva Combo (Roche)	• Holds 315 units of insulin • Bluetooth handset with remote blousing • Offers advice on carb counting • No CGM capability
Tandem t:slim X2	**Control IQ technology**: • Automatically adjusts insulin levels based on continuous glucose monitoring (CGM) readings • Delivers automatic correction boluses (up to one an hour) to help prevent hyperglycemia • Includes optional settings for Sleep Activity or Exercise Activity that adjust the range of treatment values • Uses Dexcom CGM integration **Basal IQ Technology** • Predicts and helps prevent hypoglycemic events by turning insulin deliver on and off every 5 min. It can turn insulin delivery on and off as often as every 5 min • Uses Dexcom CGM integration
Omnipod	• Tubeless sensor-augmented insulin pump • Integration with Dexcom CGM • Fully waterproof • Insulin "pods" have a lifetime of 72 h
V-Go insulin pump	• Disposable patch pump which provides both basal and prandial insulin • Used with only rapid-acting insulin • No connectivity with GM • Three available sizes which provide 0.83 μ/h (20 units of daily insulin), 1.25 μ/h (30 units of insulin), or 1.67 μ/h (40 units of insulin) • Patient can activate additional prandial or correction insulin delivery • Pump must be removed prior to undergoing an MRI
CeQur Simplicity	• Insulin "patch" which delivers ONLY prandial insulin without injections • Patch worn for 3 days • Holds up to 200 units of Humalog or Novolog insulin • Clicking (activating) the side buttons on the patch will deliver 2 units of insulin per click • CGM integration not available • Useful for patients with type 2 diabetes on multiple daily insulin injections who tend omit prandial insulin doses

[62]. The currently popular insulin pump models on the global market are Medtronic MiniMed, OmniPod (Insulet), T:Slim (Tandem), DANA R (SOOIL), Cellnovo, Accu-Chek Solo Micropump (Roche), and Ypsomed [63]. Patients with type 2 diabetes may benefit from use of the disposable V-GO insulin pumps and an injection free prandial insulin delivery patch from CeQur [6, 7].

As diabetes technologies continue to undergo rapid advancement, utilization rates are increasing across many national registries, particularly for devices related to glucose monitoring and insulin delivery [8]. Incorporating devices such as insulin pumps and continuous glucose monitors (CGM) into diabetes management helps persons with diabetes reduce their risk of treatment emergent hypoglycemia while improving HbA1c and time in range (TIR) [9]. In 2021, the American Association of Clinical Endocrinologist strongly encouraged clinicians to utilize technology for their patients with diabetes [10]. All patients with diabetes should have access to continuous glucose sensors, insulin pumps, and applications. AACE also recommended that clinicians access data beyond just assessing A1C. Using interstitial glucose monitoring patients should target a time in range (70–180 mg/dL) of 70% with less than 4% of sensor readings below 70 mg/dL. Additionally, glycemic variability (GV) should be assessed and minimized. Glycemic variability increased ones risk of developing hypoglycemia and long-term diabetes-related complications [11].

The use of sensor-automated insulin delivery (AID) systems has modernized the treatment of patients with diabetes. Patients using AID integrate the use of CGM, a blood glucose control algorithm, and an insulin delivery device such as a pump or a smart pen. Plasma glucose values are constantly fluctuating based on activities such as eating, sleeping, exercising, traveling, and illness. AID systems adjust the delivery of insulin every 5 min based on a glucose prediction algorithm. As insulin levels rise, the insulin pump will provide an automated correction dose. Likewise, insulin delivery will be paused when interstitial glucose levels are rapidly declining or if treatment emergent hypoglycemia is predicted [12]. Figure 1.1 depicts the efficacy of AID in the management of patients with type 1 diabetes.

In January 2023, Roy's CGM download demonstrated that on a typical day, blood glucose levels are under near-perfect control (Fig. 1.2). When asked, "What do you think of this automated insulin delivery technology," Roy placed his hands around his face and began to cry. "Back in 1965 I dreamed that I would have access to some magical treatment. I was so scared for my future. Now I have what I need to survive and live life to its fullest. Doctor, you have given me the gift of life. I could never thank you enough for everything you have done for me."

Bob is a rocket scientist. He works for NASA in Pasadena, California. Bob was responsible for designing the Mars Rover which is still active on that planet's surface. Bob also has had poorly controlled type 2 diabetes for 10 years. His HbA1c is 9.1%, and he has clinical evidence of microvascular complications including diabetic kidney disease, neuropathy, and retinopathy. On his initial visit to his new primary care physician, Bob, age 62, was onboarded with a freestyle libre sensor. Following a 1 h warm up period, interstitial glucose levels were streaming to his cell phone every minute of every day (1440 glucose readings daily and 20,160 every

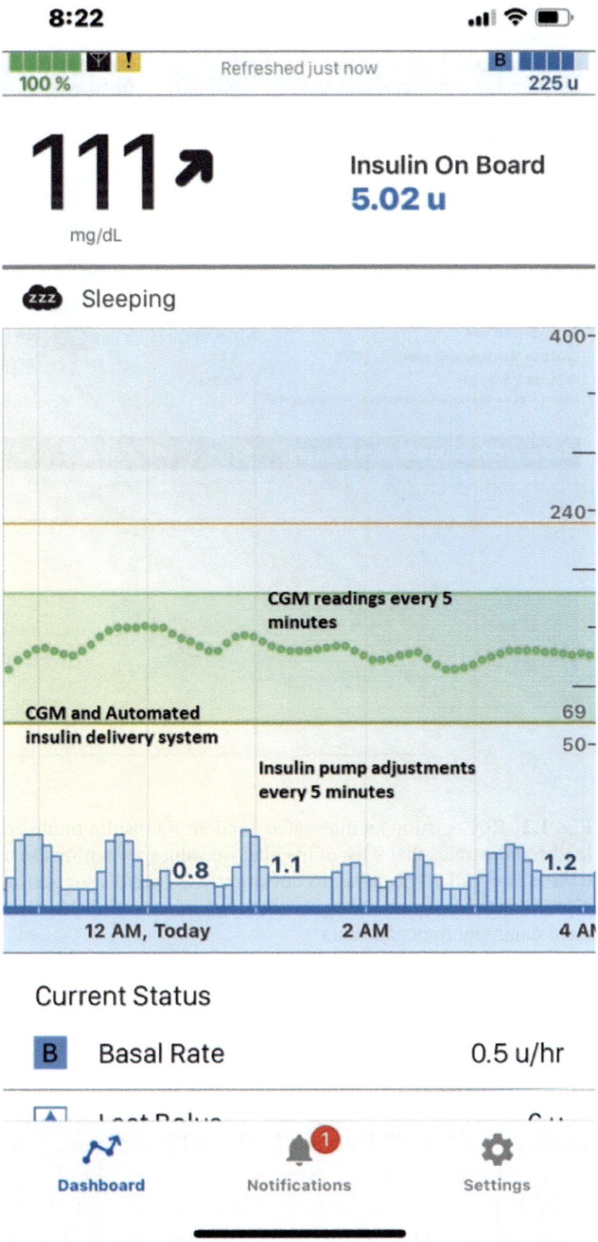

Fig. 1.1 With automated insulin delivery the continuous glucose monitor and insulin pump allows for near-perfect glycemic control. The upper graph shows the patient's interstitial glucose levels. The lower bar graph demonstrates the changes in the pump's insulin delivery every 5 min. As glucose levels rise, so does the rate of insulin deliver from the pump and vice versa. This technology reduces the likelihood of experiencing treatment emergent hypoglycemia

2 weeks). Bob returned for an unscheduled visit after just 1 week of sensor wear demanding to see his doctor. He brought with him reams of glucose data including time in range, glycemic variability, glucose management indicator (which estimates his anticipated HbA1C) as well as charts and graphs that he personally developed.

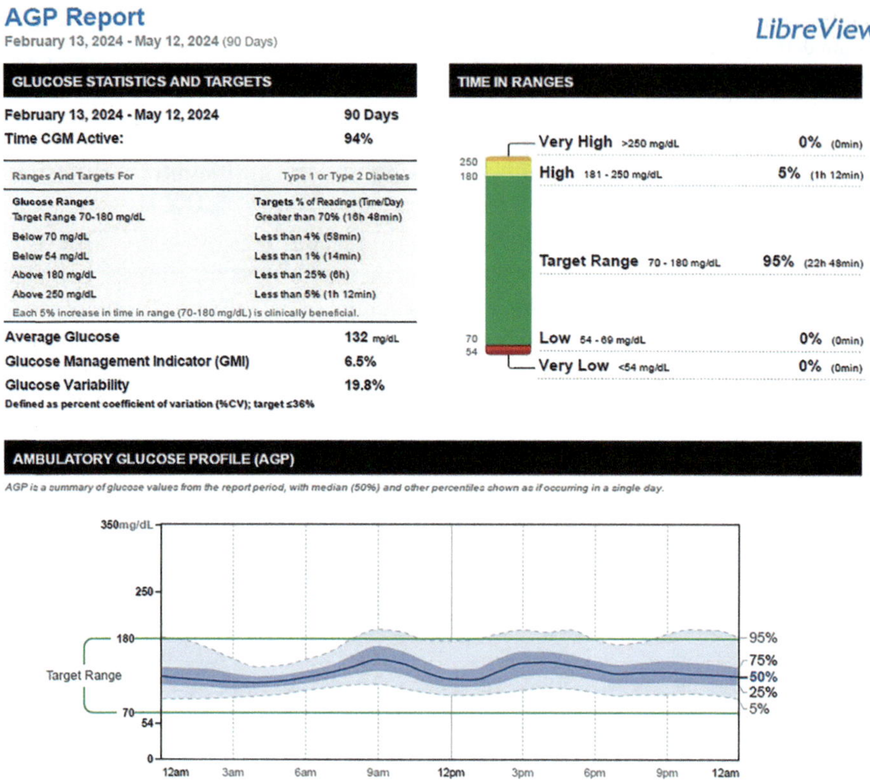

Fig. 1.2 Roy is using an integrated Tandem IQ insulin pump and a Dexcom 6 CGM. This download demonstrates that 93% of his glucose values are within the target range of 70–180 mg/dL with <1% <70 mg/dL. The standard deviation is 36 mg/dL suggesting that he is experiencing minimal glycemic variability on a daily basis. Glycemic variability increases one's risk of developing treatment emergent hypoglycemia

Bob showed his colored pie and bar charts to the doctor which included hazard ratios and *p*-values. The recently downloaded stack of roughly 200 pages of data weighed closed to 5 lbs. After quickly glancing over these charts, plots, graphs, and advanced statistical analyses, the physician asked, "Bob…what exactly are you showing me here?" Bob smiled broadly and said, "Doctor, for the first time in my life I just found out that exercise lowers my blood sugars!" Did you know that?

In 2016, the management of diabetes was quite simple. The American Diabetes Association [13] recommended that patients with type 2 diabetes start metformin. (In 3 months if the HbA1C was above 7% start a sulfonylurea. If, after three additional months the HbA1C was above target, just start a thiazolidinedione. 1 year after initiating treatment with metformin, patients with elevated HbA1C levels should be started on insulin. With the use of technology, our patients with diabetes can be treated successfully to their glycemic targets within 2–12 weeks. Patients can be assessed remotely or data can simply be downloaded at the time of each office visit. Patients can share their data with family members. The use of CGM in children means that parents do not have to awaken their kids at 3 am to perform a finger stick. Instead, CGM can alert the patient and family members to treatment emergent hypoglycemia.

Incorporation of technology for the management of our patients with diabetes is an essential part of primary and specialty care. Patients with chronic metabolic diseases such as diabetes, hypertension, hyperlipidemia, obesity, major depression, sleep apnea, kidney disease must be treated successfully to their prescribed metabolic and targets. Employing the approved technological advances available today will allow our patients to live life to the fullest. Additionally, the use of advanced technology should be addressed within the primary care setting in which 90% of all patients with diabetes are managed [14]. Readers of this book will experience and learn about the excitement our patients feel when introduced to these life-altering strategies.

References

1. Entmacher PS, Marks HH. Diabetes in 1964. A world survey. Diabetes. 1965;74:212–23. IDF Diabetes Atlas. https://diabetesatlas.org/. Accessed 1/20/23
2. Secrest AM, Washington RE, Orchard TJ. Mortality in type 1 diabetes. In: Cowie CC, Casagrande SS, Menke A, et al., editors. Diabetes in America. 3rd ed. Bethesda (MD): National Institute of Diabetes and Digestive and Kidney Diseases (US); 2018. Chapter 35. Available from: https://www.ncbi.nlm.nih.gov/books/NBK567986/.
3. Zylke JW, DeAngelis CD. Pediatric chronic diseases—stealing childhood. JAMA. 2007;297:2765–6.
4. Lipska KJ, Ross JS, Wang Y, et al. National Trends in US hospital admissions for hyperglycemia and hypoglycemia among medicare beneficiaries, 1999 to 2011. AMA Intern Med. 2014;174(7):1116–24. https://doi.org/10.1001/jamainternmed.2014.1824.
5. Fry A. Insulin delivery device technology 2012: where are we after 90 years? J Diabetes Sci Technol. 2012;6(4):947–53. https://doi.org/10.1177/193229681200600428.
6. Grunberger G, Rosenfeld CR, Bode BW, et al. Effectiveness of V-Go for patients with type 2 diabetes in a real-world setting: a prospective observational study. Drugs Real World Outcomes. 2020;7(1):31–40. (Comparing Patch vs Pen Bolus Insulin Delivery in Type 2 Diabetes Using Continuous Glucose Monitoring Metrics and Profiles)
7. Bergenstal RM, Johnson ML, Aroda VR, et al. J Diabetes Sci Technol. 2022;16(5):1167–73. https://doi.org/10.1177/19322968211016513.
8. Sherwood JS, Russell SJ, Putman MS. New and emerging technologies in type 1 diabetes. Endocrinol Metab Clin N Am. 2020;49(4):667–78. https://doi.org/10.1016/j.ecl.2020.07.006.
9. Umpierrez GE, Klonoff DC. Diabetes technology update: use of insulin pumps and continuous glucose monitoring in the hospital. Diabetes Care. 2018;41(8):1579–89. https://doi.org/10.2337/dci18-0002.
10. Grunberger G, Sherr J, Allende M, et al. AACE Guideline. American Association of Clinical Endocrinology Clinical Practice Guideline: the use of advanced technology in the management of persons with diabetes mellitus. Endocr Pract. 2021;27:505–37.
11. Ceriello A, Monnier L, Owens D. Glycaemic variability in diabetes: clinical and therapeutic implications. Lancet Diabetes Endocrinol. 2019;7(3):221–30. https://doi.org/10.1016/S2213-8587(18)30136-0.

12. Gimenez M, Conget I, Oliver N. Automated insulin delivery systems: today, tomorrow and user requirements. J Diabetes Sci Technol. 2021;15(6):1252–7.
13. American Diabetes Association. Standards of medical care in diabetes–2006. Diabetes Care. 2006;29(Suppl. 1):S4–S42. https://doi.org/10.2337/diacare.29.s1.06.s4.
14. Introduction to diabetes. In: Unger Jeff, editor. Diabetes management in primary care. Philadelphia, PA: Lippincott, Williams and Wilkins; 2007. p. 1–42.

Chapter 2
Overview of Currently Available Insulin Delivery Systems

Hayley Fried

Insulin Delivery Via Subcutaneous Route

Vial and Syringe

For the first 50 years following the discovery of insulin, injection via a vial and syringe was the only means for insulin delivery. In 1924, Becton Dickinson and Company (BD) launched the first syringe designed specifically for the injection of insulin [6]. The original large, glass, and reusable syringes were cumbersome, requiring proper sterilization techniques to prevent infection and having to sharpen the needles prior to each use. In 1954, BD developed the first disposable, glass syringe called the BD Hypak. In 1955, the first all plastic syringe (Monoject™, Roehr Products, Inc.) was created [7]. Notable advancements in the 1960s included BDs 1-mL Luer-Lock insulin syringe available with either a detachable or permanently attached needle and the widespread availability of disposable plastic syringes [7, 8]. Over the years, many advancements in syringes have been made, including the development of disposable plastic syringes, reduced plunger force, multiple barrel capacities, unit markings along the side of the syringe, and different needle gauges/lengths [7]. In 2016, the FDA approved an insulin syringe created specifically for U-500 insulin, given the dosing errors that arose from using a U-100 syringe to dose U-500 insulin [9].

The most common syringe sizes currently available on the market are 1 mL, 0.5 mL, and 0.3 mL with barrel capacities of 30 units, 50 units, and 100 units, respectively. In contrast to the needle lengths of early syringes, which ranged from 19 to 26 mm and posed a risk of intramuscular injections, the most common needle

H. Fried (✉)
Northwell Health, New York, NY, USA
e-mail: hfried1@northwell.edu

S. Fishman (ed.), *Advances in Diabetes Technology*, Contemporary Endocrinology, https://doi.org/10.1007/978-3-031-75352-7_2

lengths used today are 5 mm, 6 mm, and 8 mm [10]. One of the most commonly used needles was created by BD in 2012, called the BD Veo insulin syringe, which uses an UltraFine 6 mm needle. Its popularity is attributed to the design of the syringe, including the small diameter of the needle, which allows for decreased pain and reduced plunger force needed to administer insulin [10, 11].

Although still commercially available today, there are many drawbacks of vial syringe as means of injecting insulin, including inaccurate dosing, immense training required for patient, needing to carry several materials, and long preparation time [12], have caused many patients to seek other means of insulin delivery.

Insulin Pens

Although insulin pens do not address all limitations of insulin delivery as seen with vial and syringe, such as needle phobia, psychological impact, and needing multiple injections per day, the simplicity, flexibility, accuracy of delivering small doses of insulin, portability, decreased time to administer insulin, and reduced pain, have led to broader social acceptance, making insulin pens more favorable [13–16]. Given ease of insulin pents, patients' perceptions of insulin gradually improved, and compliance improved [15]. Since their introduction, there have been immense advancements in insulin pens that have made them one of the mainstays of insulin delivery methods today.

In comparison to vial and syringe which uses separate entities, an insulin pen is one unit composed of three components: an insulin cartridge (prefilled (disposable pen) or replaceable (reusable/durable pen)), a needle, and the injection button. Prefilled disposable insulin pens simplify the process of injections by removing the insulin cartridge loading step. Given that insulin adsorbs onto the plastic surface of prefilled pens over a period of time and a precise concentration can be accomplished via proper mixing, the dose accuracy and blood glucose stability between insulin cartridge changes are increased [17].

Among the first-generation insulin pens, the most widely used include multiple generations of the reusable NovoPen (Novo Nordisk) and Allstar (Sanofi), and the disposable Flextouch (Novo Nordisk), Humalog Pen and Kwikpen (Eli Lily). In 1985, Novo Nordisk manufactured the first type of reusable insulin pen called the NovoPen, and in 1989, the first prefilled disposable pen, called Novolet. The NovoPen family, created by Novo Nordisk, includes multiple generations of reusable pens, with each new generation's goal to continue to increase innovation. The NovoPen 2, released in 1988, allowed for a maximum dose of 36 units and featured 2 unit dosing increments, capability to set the dose prior to injection, and display the previously administered dose [18]. The NovoPen 3 released in 1992 increased the maximum dose to 70 units, had push button to release the insulin dose, and allowed resetting of the insulin dose to prevent insulin wasting [19]. The NovoPen 1.5 released in 1996 stored less insulin, therefore was shorter and improved portability. In 1999, NovoPen 3 Demi allowed for half unit dose increments, thus improved precise dosing administration of insulin. In 2003, the first pen was developed specifically for the pediatric population, called the NovoPen Junior. The NovoPen 4 launched in 2005 reduced the injection force needed, increased the font size on the display screen, ensured doses greater than amount of insulin remaining in the cartridge could not be dialed, and had auditory confirmatory dosing clicks [18]. In 2001, Novo Nordisk released the prefilled insulin pen called the FlexPen which featured an end-of-dose confirmation click, large dose display, and color coding to differentiate insulin types (thus, decreased incidental injection of long-acting versus short-acting insulin). The disposable pens by Eli Lily (KwikPen) and Sanofi (SoloStar) were launched in 2007 and 2008, respectively. In 2007, Eli Lily launched HumaPen Luxura HD, which was a reusable insulin pen that had the capability of delivering half unit dosing increments [20]. In 2011, the FlexPen was replaced with FlexTouch which provided increased accuracy and ease of use over its predecessors via spring-loaded injection mechanism (low injection force needed). Given these features that led to ease of use, it was preferred compared to other comparative insulin pens [21]. In 2012, AllStar reusable pen designed by Sanofi, was created specifically for children in India to ensure international standards were met [22]. Features of this insulin pen included easy-to-see display window for dosing, dose arrows on both sides of the insulin pen, push button to release the insulin dose, audible clicks with each unit of insulin delivered, and resetting of insulin doses to prevent insulin wasting. In 2017, the Junior Kwikpen® was available on the market, a prefilled insulin pen that allowed for half units of insulin to be administered. The Junior Kwikpen® was lighter and smaller compared to the other half unit insulin pens available on the market. In 2015, the United States Food and Drug Administration (FDA) approved higher concentration insulin pens. Concentrated insulins deliver the same dose of insulin in less volume, which are appropriate to use in insulin-resistant patients using high insulin doses. Concentrated insulin pens currently available include U-500 (Kwikpen, Humalin R®, Eli Lily), U-300 glargine (Solostar Toujeo®, Sanofi), U-200 degludec (FlexTouch, Tresiba®, Novo Nordisk), and U-200 lispro (Kwikpen Humalog®, Eli Lily) insulin. The currently available first-generation insulin pens with specialized features including multiple sized cartridges, dialing backward without wasting insulin, smaller dose increments, reduced force requirement to perform an injection, and audible clicks with each dose given, have allowed for individualization of patient management by choosing devices based on needs of patient and ease-of-use for diabetics.

In 2007, Eli Lily launched the first "smart pen" called HumaPen MEMOIR, which has memory capability to store the date, time, and amount of previous insulin doses given. In 2010, the NovoPen Echo, created for pediatric patients, was released, and was the first insulin pen that combined the half unit dosing increments with memory function (dose and time elapsed since prior injection). The NovoPen 5, released in 2015, created for the elderly population, included the design of the NovoPen 4 with the memory function of the NovoPen Echo.

One of the most advanced insulin pens currently available on the market are "connected pens," which have the capability to automatically transmit data such as the date, time, and the amount of insulin dosages administered to other applications.

They also contain built-in calculators to aid in proper insulin dosage. Given the two models of insulin pens, disposable and reusable, different technology has emerged for both unique pen types. For disposable insulin pens, there are devices such as insulin caps that attach to the pen and are able to track and submit the data. For reusable pens, companies have created built-in wireless communication capabilities to track data. Connected pen technology has allowed for sharing of information on digital platforms between members of the multidisciplinary management team and communication with other diabetes care technology.

In 2017, the FDA approved the InPen ™, created by Companion Medical, a startup company which was acquired by Medtronic in 2020. It is a Bluetooth-enabled, reusable insulin pen that connects to a smartphone application which keeps track of previous insulin doses given, recommends insulin doses, and allows users to record recent blood sugars, to set up reminders for specific dosing times, and send reports to health care providers [23]. It is compatible with rapid-acting insulin U-100 Humalog (Eli Lilly) and Novolog (Novo Nordisk) [24]. Although compatible with Dexcom's continuous glucose monitor, in 2020, Medtronic integrated InPen ™ and the Guardian Connect ™ continuous glucose monitor, which has allowed users integrate glucose value trends and insulin dosing, without any time lag [23].

In November 2022, Eli Lilly launched their first connected insulin pen system, called the Tempo® Personalized Diabetes Management Platform. FDA approved the system for DM1 and DM2, and is composed of the Tempo Smart Button®, TempoSmart™ application, and Tempo Pen®. The Tempo Smart Button® is a reusable device that attaches to the disposable Tempo Pen® and transmits data wirelessly to the application, called TempoSmart™. The application was developed in partnership with Welldoc® and has the ability to record insulin dosing and share information to health care providers with ease. Other advanced features of the TempoSmart™ insulin pen include users to be able to set medication reminders, ability to integrate with Dexcom continuous glucose monitoring, and compatibility with other devices, such as Fitbit®, Garmin®, Google Fit®, and the Apple Health application [25].

Other connected pens currently available include ESYSTA (created by Emperra) [26], NovoPen 6 and NovoPen Echo Plus (created by Novo Nordisk), [27, 28], and Pendiq 2.0 (created by Pendiq). Many studies have reported patient preference of smart pens over their previous insulin delivery method [29–33].

Although there are some drawbacks to insulin pens compared to vial and syringe as means of insulin delivery, including mechanical complexity and affordability, there are many advantages. The use of insulin pen devices have improved patient's quality of life by increasing lifestyle flexibility, improving social acceptability, convenience of injecting insulin, and reducing pain [34]. They also allow for ease of administration for patients with vision impairments and dexterity issues [21]. Studies have shown improved patient adherence with diabetes regimen with use of insulin pens versus vial and syringe [35, 36]. Given the high trend towards increased usage of smart insulin pens, in North America alone, it is projected to have a continuous annual growth rate of 26.7% by the year 2027 [37].

Injection Port

The mainstay of treatment of insulin-dependent diabetes utilizes subcutaneous injection of insulin. A study conducted in the United States by Karter et al. [38] to assess barriers to insulin initiation in DM2 revealed that 13% stated injection phobia as a cause [39]. In 2016, to combat the need for multiple injections per day and needle phobia, Medtronic launched the I-Port Advance™ Injection Port system [40]. This device allows a patient to perform multiple daily subcutaneous injections without having to puncture the skin for each dose [41]. The device is a small patch that is inserted and changed every 72 hours that allows access to subcutaneous tissues via a soft flexible cannula. Patients can then insert insulin through the port rather than through the skin via a needle [42]. In a study conducted by Kahn et al., regular users had improved compliance with insulin usage, reduced diabetes-related hospitalizations, and reduced the frequency of hypoglycemia [41].

Continuous Subcutaneous Insulin Infusion

Continuous subcutaneous insulin infusion, colloquially referred to as insulin pump therapy, is a form of insulin delivery device that imitates the physiologic continuous insulin secretion (basal), intermittent larger doses of insulin (prandial insulin), and can deliver insulin needed to cover blood glucose levels above target blood glucose level range (correction). One of the many advantages of insulin pump therapy versus multiple daily injections is the ability to set personalized basal rates per hour, thus able to microadjust insulin needs more precisely compared to an injection of long-acting insulin. From its first conceptualization in 1963 by Dr. Arnold Kadish [43], and the "Biostator" created by Dr. Ernst Friedrich Pfeiffer in 1974, earlier devices proved the feasibility of closed-loop glucose control and facilitated further technological developments to what is available on the market today [44].

At its core purpose and function, insulin pumps are small devices that deliver insulin through the infusion set, which is a catheter that is inserted into subcutaneous tissue and secured to skin with adhesive. Patch pumps directly connect to the infusion set, adhere to the skin, and are controlled wirelessly through a separate remote whereas other insulin pumps utilize tubing to connect the infusion set to the insulin pump. Within insulin pumps, there are reservoirs with different reservoir capacities that store insulin. Rapid-acting insulins (lispro, aspart, and glulisine) are recommended to be used within the insulin pump. Although insulin lispro and aspart can be stored in a reservoir for up to 144 h, insulin glulisine must be replaced every 48 h due to increased risk of crystallization that can lead to occlusions [45]. Infusion sets are removed and reinserted every few days (time frame dependent on infusion set used), therefore do not require multiple daily injections. Users pre-set basal rates prior to insulin pump use. Other information, such as insulin sensitivity factor (how much one unit of insulin is expected to lower the patient's blood glucose level), target blood glucose level (blood glucose level is used to calculate the correction insulin dose), and insulin to carbohydrate ratio (how many carbohydrates one unit of insulin is expected to achieve stabilization to neither decrease nor increase current blood glucose level) can also be pre-programmed. Insulin pumps also contain a bolus calculator in which takes the current blood glucose level, target blood glucose level, insulin sensitivity factor, insulin to carbohydrate ratio, total carbohydrates eaten by insulin pump user, and insulin on board (the amount of insulin currently active from prior insulin doses) into consideration to calculate a recommended insulin dose. Temporary basal rates, which allow the user to increase or decrease the current basal rate, can also be utilized, which is useful for acute situations that warrant a change to allow for normalization of blood glucose levels, such as an acute illness or during physical activity. Some pumps allow for an extended bolus option, which delivers a portion of the short-acting insulin immediately and another portion to be extended over a longer period of time. This is advantageous to prevent delayed postprandial hyperglycemia, which can be seen in patients with gastroparesis or after high fatty content meals.

Given the implications of the Diabetes Control and Complications Trial favoring intensive insulin therapy to prevent diabetic complications, there has been immense research and advancements in insulin pump therapy, which has dramatically increased their usage. The global insulin pump market size was valued at $4.60 billion United States dollars (USD) in 2022 and is projected to grow from $5.23 billion USD in 2023 to $15.51 billion USD by 2030 [46]. The main companies that hold a major share in the insulin pump market include Medtronic Minimed, Inc., Tandem Diabetes Care, Inc., Ypsomed Holding AG, and Insulet Corporation, all of which offer their own unique features. Advancements in the field of insulin pump therapy are occurring at an astonishing rate; therefore, it is important for providers to stay up to date with current technology to properly inform patients to help manage their diabetes.

Sensor-Augmented Pump Therapy

The development of continuous glucose monitor (CGM) sensors was a major step towards the development of "closed-loop" insulin delivery systems. Sensor-augmented pump therapy integrates CGM sensor information with insulin pumps. In 2006, the FDA approved the world's first sensor-augmented pump therapy system, the Minimed™ Paradigm™ REAL-Time system that utilized CGM sensor data to communicate with insulin pumps to automatically increase or decrease the basal rate. Studies have shown reduction in hypoglycemic episodes and superior glucose level control with sensor-augmented pump therapy compared to conventional therapy [47, 48]. In 2009, Medtronic launched the MiniMed™ Veo ™ System outside of the United States, which was the world's first insulin pump with automatic low glucose insulin delivery suspension when blood glucose levels have reached a set low threshold. Several studies have shown sensor-augmented pump therapy with additional hypoglycemia auto-suspend has further reduced the rate of hypoglycemic episodes and reduce the psychological burden of the fear of nocturnal hypoglycemia [49–51]. The Automation to Simulate Pancreatic Insulin Response Trial showed that sensor-augmented insulin pump therapy with a low glucose suspend function significantly reduced nocturnal hypoglycemia without raising Hemoglobin A1C (HbA1c) [52]. In 2010, the FDA approved the next-generation Minimed™ Paradigm REAL-Time Revel™ System which incorporated predictive alerts to cue users into current blood glucose levels trends heading towards dangerous out-of-target range.

Continuous Glucose Monitoring

Although not a mode of insulin delivery, given the synergism and integration of CGM sensors and insulin pump therapy, we will briefly discuss the technology. According to the 2023 Standards of Care in Diabetes, real-time CGM or intermittently scanned CGM should be offered to individuals with DM1 or DM2 on multiple daily injections, basal insulin, or continuous subcutaneous insulin infusion who are capable of using the devices safely [5]. Unlike conventional glucose monitors that only allows for snapshot readings of blood glucose levels, CGMs are devices that allow for semi-continuous blood glucose level readings. CGMs are wearable devices that are inserted into subcutaneous tissue and extrapolate blood glucose levels from interstitial fluid glucose levels. Since FDA approval in 1999, the technology has immensely improved, including increased accuracy [53]. CGMs can be continuous or intermittently scanned. Devices can be designated as needing calibration (requiring blood glucose levels via separate blood glucose monitoring device to be taken and inserted into CGM technology system), adjunctive (to be used in addition to separate blood glucose monitoring before clinical decision-making) or non-adjunctive (devices integrated with other devices that do not need calibration). Benefits of CGM technology have been well documented across all age classes and types of diabetes. Studies have shown reductions in HbA1c levels and decreased episodes of hypoglycemia [54–57]. Studies have shown that in patients with DM1, the frequency of sensor use correlates with decreased HbA1c [54, 58]. In DM2, CGM discontinuation causes partial reversal in HbA1c and time in range, suggesting continuing CGM technology achieves the greatest outcomes [59]. In a randomized control trial designed to assess CGM technology and its effects on pregnant persons with DM1 resulted in mild improvements in HbA1c without increased risk of hypoglycemia and decreased large-for-gestational-age births, length of stay, and neonatal hypoglycemia [60].

Although there are many positive outcomes from the advancements and use of CGM technology, there are some limitations. Some downfalls of CGM monitoring include lag time of interstitial glucose levels compared to blood glucose levels, most pronounced in times of rapid blood glucose level changes. Irritant and allergic contact dermatitis secondary to the adhesive used has also been documented [61]. There are many medications that interfere with the sensor, leading to discrepancies in actual blood glucose level versus CGM readings, including lisinopril, ascorbic acid, hydroxyurea, albuterol, acetaminophen, atenolol, and red wine [62] have been documented. Steps have been taken by different CGM system manufacturers to reduce this interference. For example, Dexcom created a novel design of their CGM G6 system by adding a permselective membrane to block the diffusion of acetaminophen to the electrode surface, thereby minimizing its interference [63, 64].

Do-It-Yourself Artificial Pancreas Systems

Amidst all of the positive outcome announcements of the upcoming closed-loop systems, patients with diabetes were eager to begin using the technology. However, given the immense process before commercialization of a product, such as clinical trials, regulatory procedures, and FDA approval, patients became increasingly impatient, thus sparking the #WeAreNotWaiting movement in 2013 to develop open-sourced diabetes management systems in. During the time period to develop and commercialize FDA-approved systems, tech savvy people developed their own closed-loop systems, referred to as "Do-it-yourself artificial pancreas systems" (DIY-APS) and shared their programs online for other users. There are three types of DIY-APS: OpenAPS, AndroidAPS, and Loop. Each of these systems uses unauthorized algorithms to collect and analyze data on blood glucose levels (via continuous glucose monitors), insulin, and carbohydrate intake to predict future glucose trends to calculate insulin doses. This information is then sent to the insulin pump to adjust insulin delivery. Information is continuously fed back into the system where it is analyzed to make future adjustments [65]. Although these systems do not have FDA approval, health care professionals should be aware of these systems to keep patients safe who are using them [5].

Closed-Loop Systems

The newest technological advancements in insulin pump therapy include closed-loop automated insulin delivery systems that integrate insulin pump therapy and continuous glucose monitor data to adjust insulin delivery based on sensor-derived glucose levels to mimic physiologic insulin delivery. These systems are composed of a continuous glucose monitor sensor, an insulin pump, and an algorithm to analyze data between the two devices to calculate required insulin dosing. This technology has integrated low glucose suspension, basal delivery adjustments, and correction boluses. However, manual entry of carbohydrates consumed to calculate mealtime boluses must be entered. In 2013, the FDA approved the Minimed™ 530G with Enlite™, the first system that incorporated low glucose suspension function that automatically halted insulin delivery when a certain trend was predicted. Medtronic introduced the Minimed 640G system in 2015 which in addition to new technological advancements from the model prior, integrated insulin tracking, bolus progress bar, and predictive battery life.

In 2017, the FDA-approved Minimed™ 670G, the world's first hybrid closed-loop system. This system's main objective was to maximize blood glucose level time in range by automatically adjusting basal rates. The pump has two modes, a manual mode which allowed the insulin pump to function as a traditional insulin pump, and an automated mode, which when paired with a continuous glucose monitor, had auto-predicted low glucose suspend and auto basal insulin adjustments [66]. Studies have shown reduction in HbA1c [67–69], reduced risk of exercise-related hypoglycemia [70], and psychosocial benefits [71, 72]. OmniPod® is the most prominent patch pump currently available on the market. The OmniPod® Insulin Management System was designed by Insulet Corporation and received FDA approval in 2003. Omnipod DASH® Insulin Management System gained FDA approval in 2018 which featured a new sleek, touchscreen personal diabetes manager (PDM) with the food database Calorie King built in to allow users to search foods for proper carbohydrate counting. Instead of a built-in freestyle glucometer within the PDM as prior models, the new generation came with a Contour Next One stand-alone glucometer. The Omnipod DASH ® is compatible with mobile applications that sync the insulin pump and, if used, CGM information onto a single portal that users can share information with health care providers.

Tandem t:slim x2 with control-IQ technology was FDA approved in 2019 with its main objective to reduce glucose level variability by automatically decreasing, stopping, or increasing basal insulin if CGM readings are predicted to be out of range [73]. In addition, it also has the capability to deliver automatic correction boluses to prevent hyperglycemia. Studies comparing Control-IQ and sensor-augmented pump therapy showed increased time in targeted range (70–180 mg/dL), reduced hypoglycemia episodes, and reduction in HbA1c [67].

In 2022, Insulet launched the fifth-generation Omnipod® 5 Automated Insulin Delivery System. The system connects the pod with a CGM and uses the Smartadjust™ algorithm to use CGM readings every 5 min to predict trends and adjust insulin doses and basal rate accordingly. This system has been shown to prevent hyperglycemia and hypoglycemia. Another unique feature is the ability to use a smartphone rather than a PDM to administer insulin.

In 2022, Ypsomed, Abbott, and CamDiab announced their partnership to develop an automated insulin delivery system utilizing the Ypsomed's mylife YpsoPump with Abbott's FreeStyle's Libre 3 CGM sensor and CamDiab's CamAPS FX mobile application to be launched in Europe. Currently, users can choose between Freestyle's Libre 3 (sensor sends data every minute) and Dexcom's CGM (sensor sends data every 3 minutes) in which data is sent to CamAPS FX application to adjust insulin delivery settings via the pump to maintain glucose readings within the target range [74]. In the hopes of commercializing their product in the United States, Ypsomed announced their partnership with Eli Lilly in November, 2020. However, in December 2022, Eli Lilly discontinued the partnership, wanting to focus more of their diabetes management efforts on their connected pen technology. Ypsomed is still planning to submit its YpsoPump system to the FDA and commercialize the system with a new partner in the United States [25].

In January of 2023, Tidepool Loop, a nonprofit organization, became the first "do-it-yourself" open-source automated insulin delivery system to gain FDA approval. This software includes a CGM, the Tidepool Loop algorithm, and an alternate controller-enabled insulin pump. The application contains a "pre-meal preset" mode, in which user sets desired blood glucose range at mealtime to decrease blood glucose levels that can occur with improper insulin dosing at meal time. Users can adjust the amount of insulin before or after meal by entering estimated amount of carbohydrates into the application. The application also has expanded compatibility with devices, including the ability to be directly controlled with an Apple Watch. Unlike other automated insulin delivery systems that have exclusivity with a limited number of companies, Tidepool Loop does not have this limitation, thus allowing the user to have flexibility over what CGM and insulin pump they can use with the software [75]. In May of 2023, Embecta Corporation announced its new partnership with Tidepool Loop to develop an automated insulin deliver system for DM2. Their main focus is to create a user-friendly system to help improve outcomes for people with DM2 [76].

In 2023, Medtronic introduced the MiniMed ™ 780G system using SmartGuard™ technology with mealtime detection, which automates the adjustments of both basal and correction boluses dependent on blood glucose levels every 5 min [77]. In addition, it is the only insulin pump that is compatible with an infusion set that can be worn for up to 7 days, an extended amount of time compared to other infusion sets currently on the market. The infusion set contains advanced materials that aid in insulin preservation loss, maintain insulin flow and stability, therefore decreased risk of infusion set occlusion [78]. In the United States, Pivotal Trial Data for MiniMed™ 780G Advanced Hybrid Closed-Loop System with Automated Correction Bolus Feature reported overall time in range of 75% with overall time below range (defined as less than 70 mg/dL) as 1.8%, overnight time in range of 82% with overnight time below range of 1.5% and autocorrection contributing 22% of all bolus insulin [42].

In July 2023, Tandem announced FDA approval of the Tandem Mobi. This insulin pump features a 200-unit insulin cartridge and an on-pump button that provides an alternative to phone control for dosing insulin. It is less than half the size of the t-slim X2 insulin pump and can be worn on the body with an adhesive sleeve or with a detachable infusion set with 5-inch tubing. The pump also contains the automated insulin delivery system with Control-IQ Technology as seen with the previous model. The insulin pump allows full smartphone control through the mobile application [79].

Alternate Controller-Enabled Infusion (ACE) Pumps

Another innovation in insulin delivery technology includes the development of alternate controller-enable infusion (ACE) pumps. ACE pumps are interoperable, thus can be combined with different components that make up diabetes therapy systems, which allows users to tailor diabetes management to fit their personal needs and device preferences. Examples of different technologies in which ACE pumps can be used in conjunction with include automated insulin dosing systems, CGMs, and glucometers. In 2019, the FDA approved its first ACE pump, the t:Slim X2 insulin pump. The insulin pump can be programmed to digitally connect and automatically communicate with and receive insulin dosing commands from other diabetes management devices (such as a smart phone). The FDA established criteria, called special controls, which outline the specific requirements needed to become an ACE insulin pump. These include the accuracy and reliability of the rate and volume of insulin to be delivered by the user, the ability of the insulin pump to communicate with other diabetes management devices, and cybersecurity [80]

Although insulin delivery via multiple, intermittent injections a day can achieve euglycemia, it does not properly imitate the mechanism of the pancreas, causing variability in blood sugar readings. Compared to multiple daily insulin injections, continuous subcutaneous insulin infusion has been associated with better glycemic control [81], particularly in those with individuals with higher baseline HbA1c [82], and less variability in blood glucose concentrations, prevention in long-term complications, reduction in total insulin dose needed daily to achieve goals [83, 84], and improvement in quality of life [85]. Complications of pump therapy include pump site infection and diabetic ketoacidosis (in the setting of failed infusion sets) [86, 87].

According to a study, using the Type 1 Diabetes Exchange Clinic registry data from 2016 to 2018, the use of an insulin pump increased from 57% in 2010–2012 to 63% in 2016–2018 [88]. It has been documented that utilization of insulin pump therapy is associated with socioeconomic status, race, age, and gender. There is documented higher insulin pump usage in patients with higher socioeconomic status [89, 90] and lower usage with non-Hispanic Black, non-native English speakers, male diabetics, and the older population [88]. Causes of these disparities include preference for multiple daily injections, provider bias, cost, and insurance denial [88]. It is important for health care providers to understand social determinants of health to effectively combat disparities and to strive for equitable levels of care [91].

According to the American Diabetes Association "Standards of Care in Diabetes" released in 2023, continuous insulin pump therapy has become standard of care and should be offered to all insulin-dependent diabetes patients who are capable of using the device safely [86, 92]. Automated insulin delivery systems are preferred over non-automated pumps and insulin pen injections in people with DM1 given the advantage of lower HbA1c and reduction in severe hypoglycemia in children and adults [93].

Insulin Pumps Designed for DM2

Although initially approved for DM1, insulin pumps can now be used by insulin-dependent DM2 patients [94]. Studies have shown reduction in HbA1c, decrease total daily dose of insulin, and improved treatment satisfaction with insulin pump use in DM2 irrespective of baseline c-peptide level [95–98]. Conventional insulin pumps currently on the market have many advanced features, such as the ability to set numerous basal rates at different times and built-in bolus calculators based on carbohydrate intake. Although beneficial for the management of patients with DM1, these features are not always necessary for those with DM2 and may contribute to complex education and underutilization of insulin pumps within the DM2 population [94, 99]. Studies have shown simple insulin delivery devices reduce barriers to insulin therapy in patients with DM2 [100].

Insulin pumps specifically designed for the DM2 population include PAQ and Simplicity (both manufactured by CeQur),V-Go (manufactured byValeritas) and Omnipod GO™ (manufactured by Insulet). V-Go®, which received FDA approval in 2012, is a patch pump that requires no programming. It is available in three models which differ by the dosing of constant basal infusion (20 units, 30 units, or 40 units per day). All models allow for mealtime and correction insulin dosing in two-unit increments. It must be changed daily and is compatible with U-100 insulin. It is available in the United States [101]. PAQ, which became available to the public in 2021, is a patch pump that allows users to program the device between seven different basal rates. It allows for mealtime and correction insulin dosing in two-unit increments. It can be worn for up to 3 days, holds up to 330 units, and is compatible with U-100 insulin. It is currently only available in Europe [102]. Simplicity, which received FDA approval in 2021, is a patch pump that differs from the other patch pumps in that there is no basal rate feature. The pump's sole purpose is for mealtime and correction insulin dosing. It can be worn for up to 3 days and is compatible with U-100 insulin [103]. Omnipod GO™ which received FDA approval in 2023 (with plans for commercializing in the United States in 2024) is a patch pump that differs from the other patch pumps in that it delivers basal insulin only. It features only a Pod, which is offered in seven pre-programmed daily rates ranging from 10 to 40 units per day and operates independently from a PDM [104].

Bionic Pancreas

The bionic pancreas is a type of insulin delivery method in which utilizes two separate infusion pumps to deliver glucagon and insulin. While current closed-loop systems rely on user to input data such as basal rates, insulin sensitivity factor, and carbohydrate-to-insulin ratios upon initiation of device, the bionic pancreas determines its own settings based solely on body weight and data gathered from the CGM. Users input qualitative information at meal times, referred to as meal-announcement doses ("usual for me," "more," "less") in which the algorithm assesses the insulin need. The algorithm continually adapts to the users' needs and cannot be overridden, thus incapable of modifying insulin dosing [105]. In 2023, Beta Bionics gained FDA approval of the iLet Bionic Pancreas. This technology is the first and only automated insulin delivery system that does not require pre-set basal rates, user entered correction or carbohydrate counting, and fully automates 100% of all user insulin doses [106]. A trial in which assessed bionic pancreas use in DM1 patients for 13 weeks showed an association with greater reduction in HbA1c levels compared to the current standard of care [105].

Jet Injectors

It has been well studied that needle phobia is associated with poor glycemic control, clinical complications, psychological comorbidities, poor general well-being and health status, and increased mortality for patients [13, 107–109]. Needle-free injectors, called jet injectors, use a high pressure mechanism to allow a small stream of insulin to penetrate the epidermis to enter subcutaneous tissue with minimal tissue damage [110]. This high velocity system allows for dispersion of insulin over a larger subcutaneous area without the use of of a needle [111]. Studies have shown that administration of insulin (short- and rapid-acting) via jet injector achieved peak levels within a short time period compared to insulin pens [112–114]. Another study conducted to investigate efficacy of an insulin jet injector and an insulin pen in treatment of patients with DM2 revealed that insulin aspart administration via jet injector reduced postprandial glucose levels within a shorter time frame, compared to insulin pens [109].

Development of jet injector technology began as in the 1860s and was offered specifically for the administration of insulin in the 1940s, called Hypospray. The current insulin jet injectors on the market were released in the 1990s and are classified as disposable cartridge liquid jet injectors. Liquid jet injectors are composed of the power source (spring or compressed gas), piston, drug-loaded compartment, and nozzle. Once activated, the power source pushes the piston and rapidly increases the pressure within the drug-loaded compartment and shoots the insulin out of the nozzle at a high velocity [115]. The jet injector is able to disperse insulin into subcutaneous adipose tissue with efficiency over 90% [116]. Insujet™, acquired by Nugen Medical Devices in 2020, is a product developed by a small team of dedicated people who believe in a needle-free future for patients with chronic conditions. The development of the technology began in 2004 and received European Union market approval in 2010. The current model, the Insujet V5, is compatible with all U-100 insulins, allows 4–50 units to be given in 1 unit increments, and can be used up to 5000 times. Although it is not available in the United States, it is available in over 40 countries, has three global offices and has over 25 global partners [117].

Although jet injectors have many advantages, there has not been wide acceptance of the technology secondary to the cost, decreased efficiency with repeated use, and infection rates that were seen with vaccination administration from 1950 to

1990 with the multiuse nozzle jet injector [118, 119]. Other adverse reactions include bleeding, hematoma formation [120, 121]. Some studies have shown that they are not less painful than insulin injections [122, 123].

Insulin Delivery Via Intraperitoneal Route

Subcutaneous insulin resistance is a rare syndrome in which patients with poorly controlled glucose levels are thought to have protease-mediated insulin degradation within subcutaneous tissue [124]. To combat this, continuous intraperitoneal insulin infusion was created. Intraperitoneal insulin is directly infused into the intraperitoneal space where it is then absorbed by the capillaries of the viscera into the portal vein [124]. It takes 15 min to reach peak effect and has a more predictable effect on blood glucose levels compared to subcutaneous injection [124]. This route of administration mimics physiologic insulin release more closely than subcutaneous methods [125]. In 2000, Medtronics gained Conformité Européenne (CE) approval of the implantable insulin pump Model 2007-A, for DM1 patients unable to achieve glucose control through subcutaneous insulin delivery. The pump was inserted into the subcutaneous tissue of the lower abdomen and contained a battery that had a 7-year lifespan. The catheter attached to the pump was directed towards the direction of the liver and delivered insulin directly into the peritoneal space. The pump was controlled by an external remote control. The patient would refill the reservoir via transcutaneous means approximately every 3 months [126]. However in 2007, Medtronic discontinued the implantable insulin pump. In 2000, Accu-Check ® DiaPort system (Roche Diabetes care GmbH) was created, which is a continuous intraperitoneal insulin delivery. It consists of a small port body which is implanted into subcutaneous tissue of the abdomen, a catheter directed to the liver, and an external insulin pump (Spirit Combo insulin pump) that is connected to the port via an infusion set [127].

Compared to continuous subcutaneous insulin infusion treatment, continuous intraperitoneal insulin infusion treatment was found to have better HbA1c levels and decreased fluctuations in blood glucose levels [128]. There are many potential adverse effects of insulin delivery via intraperitoneal means. Given the invasive, operative placement of the device, surgical complications such as infection (sometimes leading to peritonitis), prolonged device-related pain, and hematoma formation occurred [129]. Other adverse effects included pump dislocation, catheter occlusion, and hardware failures (premature battery failure and pump dysfunction [129].

Insulin Delivery Via Pulmonary Route

Several exogenous, non-conventional, non-oral routes of administration have been studied, one of which is inhalation. The pulmonary route of administration is favorable given its large surface area, highly permeable membrane, high blood perfusion, and lack of mucociliary clearance [130]. Compared to subcutaneous insulin lispro, inhaled insulin had a faster onset of action and longer duration of action [131]. Given these results, inhaled insulin is best suited for prandial insulin use in patients with diabetes.

The first FDA-approved inhaled insulin product was a powdered formulation created by Pfizer, known as Exubera, which was commercially available from August 2006 to October 2007. However, only after a short period of time, it was discontinued. Broad public acceptance failure, needing for additional testing such as frequent pulmonary function testing, increased risk of hypoglycemia, high cost, and problems with its cumbersome construction were the main drivers that led to its discontinuation in 2007 [132, 133]. The withdrawal of Exubera from the market led to a cascade of pharmaceutical company halts on the research and development of inhaled insulin [134].

In June 2014, an inhaled insulin product created by Mannkind, called Afrezza, used a new type of technology, called Technosphere Inhaled Insulin which had unique pharmacokinetics/pharmacodynamics that allowed for a more rapid onset of action and shorter duration of action compared to rapid-acting insulin analogs [135]. This is still commercially available today.

Inhaled insulin advantages are most prominent when considering quality of life, such as an alternative for patients with needle phobia, ease of administration, social acceptance, and decreased pain at injection site [136]. Although it has advantages, it also has many drawbacks. Patients must undergo pre-treatment evaluation with pulmonary function testing, repeated after 6 months of inhaled insulin use, then yearly thereafter as lung safety has been questioned. Given the finite number of prefilled, predetermined insulin amounts within the cartridges, fine insulin adjustments are not possible. Patients also must still use injectable basal insulin as inhaled insulin is only for post-prandial use. Common side effects of inhaled include cough, throat irritation, and acute bronchospasm [137]. Contraindications to its use include patients with long-term lung conditions, active smokers, recently stopped smoking in last 6 months, and patients with high risk of diabetic ketoacidosis development. The drug delivery has not been studied in patients under 18 years of age and pregnant persons [137–139].

Insulin Delivery Via Oral Route

The oral route of insulin administration is a patient-friendly means of insulin delivery in which many biopharmaceutical companies are currently developing formulations. Subcutaneous insulin administered does not properly reach the liver to an appropriate degree, thus impairing postprandial glycogen storage, leading to an inability to mobilize hepatic glucose needed to counteract hypoglycemia. Formulations of oral insulin are currently under development with the hopes to enhance insulin delivery to the liver, thus facilitating hepatic carbohydrate uptake and conversion to glycogen to be stored [140]. Given that the oral route of insulin administration provides a direct route to the liver via portal circulation, side effects seen with parenteral insulin administration such as peripheral hyperinsulinemia, weight gain, and hypoglycemia can potentially be avoided [141]. Certain properties of insulin have made the development of oral insulin a challenge. Insulin is a peptide hormone, in which has low permeability through gastrointestinal epithelial cells given its hydrophobic nature, has a large molecular size, and is inactivated by proteolytic enzymes within the gastrointestinal system, resulting in poor bioavailability [142, 143]. To improve bioavailability, multiple formulations have been trialed, including co-administration with absorption enhancers [144], co-administration with enzyme inhibitors [144], chemical modification [145], and carrier molecules (such as liposomes, micelles, microspheres and nanoparticles, and polymeric hydrogels) to serve as a vehicle for insulin delivery [146–148]. Multiple clinical trials are still ongoing to investigate the efficacy of oral insulin, in which a few are listed below in more detail.

Absorption Enhancers

In 2006, Oramed Pharmaceuticals, Inc., a clinical-stage pharmaceutical company focused on the development of oral drug delivery systems, began development of their orally ingestible insulin capsule, referred to as ORMD-08081. Their most recent FDA-approved study is ORA-D-013, which evaluated the efficacy and safety of ORMD-0801, their oral insulin capsule with absorption enhancers, protease inhibitors, enteric coating, and emulsifier, in subjects with DM2 with inadequate glycemic control on one to three oral glucose-lowering agents. The primary endpoint of the study was to compare the efficacy of ORMD-0801 compared to placebo in improving glycemic control via assessing the mean change from baseline HbA1c at 26 weeks. The secondary endpoint was to assess efficacy of ORMD-0801 compared to placebo via the mean change from baseline in fasting plasma glucose at 26 weeks [149]. Although the ORA-D-013 study showed promise, in January 2023, Phase 3 results were release and it was concluded that the trial did not meet its primary or secondary clinical endpoints [150]. In May 2023, Oramed announced that its partner, Hefei Tianhui Biotechnology Co. Ltd., successfully completed its Phase 3 trials of oral insulin in DM2 in China. This success has allowed them to move a step forward to commercialization and is pending regulatory approval. Although discouraged from results from ORMD-0801 Phase 3 trial, Oramed may reconsider ways to move forward with their oral insulin product in the future [151].

Enzyme Inhibitors

The biopharmaceutical company Diabetology Limited, a subsidiary of Proxima Concepts Limited headquartered in the United Kingdom, dedicated to the development of oral drugs for the treatment of diabetes, created Capsulin™, an oral insulin capsule formulation. Capsulin™ is an enteric-coated capsule containing a dry powder formulation of regular human insulin and other compounds to protect the insulin from degradation, facilitate transport, and uptake by gut epithelial cells. The capsule passes through the stomach and the contents are released into the small intestine, absorbed by cells within the gastrointestinal tract, and travel directly to the liver via the portal vein. Capsulin™ is currently undergoing clinical trials. Phase 2b was conducted from January 2019 to July 2020 to evaluate the safety and efficacy of Capsulin™ in subjects with uncontrolled DM2 on Metformin. The study met its primary and secondary clinical endpoints which were to observe statistically significant changes from baseline HbA1c (greater than 0.5%) and fasting plasma glucose level (within the 150 iu BD group) with the use of Capsulin™. Other results showed a statistically significant reduction in low-density lipoprotein cholesterol, total cholesterol, and triglycerides with the use of Capsulin™. There was no increased risk of hypoglycemic incidents with Capsulin™ compared to metformin [152]. Although still under investigation, the positive results from the clinical trials show promise in commercialization in the near future.

Chemical Modification

Biocon is a biopharmaceutical company that developed an oral ultra-rapid-acting prandial insulin formulation, called Tregopil. Tregopil is a recombinant human insulin that underwent chemical modification to enhance bioavailability. The study enrolled DM2 subjects actively prescribed metformin and insulin glargine tested the efficacy and safety of Tregopil compared to insulin aspart. The results of the Phase 2/3 study published in 2022 did not meet its clinical endpoints. There was no observed improvement in baseline HbA1C and although Tregopil's early postprandial effects were comparable to insulin aspart, its late postprandial effects were inferior [145].

Carrier Molecules

Oshadi Drug Administration Limited developed an oral insulin that utilizes carrier molecules, called Oshadi Icp, to enhance bioavailability. The drug contains a combination of insulin, proinsulin, and c-peptide. It is currently under clinical investigation for use for DM1 patients. Phase 1 of the clinical trial demonstrated that use of oral drug with subcutaneous insulin lowers plasma glucose within 7 hours post oral drug use and decreased total daily dose of subcutaneous insulin required. Phase 2 of the clinical trial demonstrated a significant reduction in the subcutaneous insulin dose to carbohydrate intake with oral insulin drug use [153]. Currently, Oshadi Icp is undergoing further clinical trials.

Diasome Pharmaceuticals, Inc., a biopharmaceutical company focused on the development of cell-targeted therapies for treating diabetes and obesity, developed a hepatic-directed vesicle (HDV) insulin to be used in conjunction with subcutaneous insulin. Insulin binds the HDV complex and targets the liver via receptors. The ISLE-1 study demonstrated that in DM1 subjects with HbA1c greater than 8.5%, the use of HDV-lispro decreased time spent with hypoglycemia and lowered Hba1c (compared to subjects on lispro alone which had the same reduction in HbA1c with increased time spent with hypoglycemia, in which they attributed to patient hesitation to alter bolus insulin dosing in the setting of blinded drug and blinded continuous glucose monitor data). Subjects with HbA1c less than 8.5% did not have reductions in Hba1c or time spent with hypoglycemia with HDV-lispro. The OPTI-1 study was designed to ascertain the benefit of HDV-insulin in DM1 patients with HbA1c <8.5% with unblinded continuous glucose monitor data and a mandated increase in bolus: basal insulin ratio via a reduction in basal insulin at time of initiation of HDV-lispro administration [154]. Results demonstrated the addition of HDV to mealtime lispro decreased time spent with hypoglycemia, with most prominent reduction in nocturnal hypoglycemia. Thus, proving that increased delivery of insulin to the liver reduces the risk of hypoglycemia [154].

Emisphere Technologies, Inc., a drug delivery company created to develop formulations to improve oral formulations of poorly permeable active pharmaceutical ingredients, was acquired by Novo Nordisk in 2020. With this acquisition, they obtained ownership of the Eligen® SNAC technology. This technology enables drug therapies to be given via tablet form by the addition of absorption enhancing molecules to be able to transport large peptides/proteins across gastrointestinal epithelial cell membranes [155]. An example of the success of the technology is Rybelsus®, an oral semaglutide approved by the FDA in 2019.

Insulin Delivery Via Buccal Route

Buccal deliver of insulin offers a potential noninvasive means of insulin delivery. The buccal surface has many advantages for insulin absorption, such as high density of blood vessels, large surface area, and direct access to the jugular veins to bypass first pass metabolism [141, 156, 157]. Two clinical trials to investigate buccal insulin delivery were discontinued. Oral-lyn™ , a liquid formulation developed by Generex Biotechnology used delivered micellar oral insulin spray via a device called a RapidMist™ system [158]. However, the clinical trial was discontinued in India due to lack of clinical efficacy [158]. MonoSol Rx (PharmaFilm®Z) and Midatech partnered to create MSL-001, a mucoadhesive polymeric film bound to glycan-coated gold nanoparticles to deliver mucosal insulin, however was discontinued due to low insulin bioavailability.

Insulin Delivery Via Transplantation

Pancreatic transplantation therapy was created with the main goals to increase the quality of life of patients with DM1, restore endogenous insulin secretion to create independence from exogenous insulin needs, and to halt the progression of diabetic complications [159]. In 1966, the first whole-pancreatic transplant was conducted in conjunction with a kidney transplant on a patient with uremia and DM1 at the University of Minnesota Hospital [160]. In the mid-1990s, the use of tacrolimus and mycophenolate to combat organ transplant rejection and advances in surgical technique improved patient and graft survival and consequently increased the number of pancreatic transplants performed [161]. According to the International Pancreas Transplant Registry between 1966 and 2020, a total of 63,871 pancreatic transplants were performed [162]. Patient survival rate at 1 year is greater than 96% in all three categories of transplantation and pancreas graft survival is >90% for simultaneous pancreas and kidney and >86% for solitary transplants [162]. Although DM2 was once considered a contraindication to pancreatic transplantation, studies have shown positive outcomes in certain patients [163, 164]. Pancreatic transplantation is currently still the only method to obtain long-term insulin dependence and euglycemia [162].

There are three main modalities for whole-pancreatic organ transplantation: simultaneous pancreatic and kidney transplant, pancreatic transplant after renal transplant, and pancreatic transplant alone [161]. Although a transplant can be seen as curative, given the side effects and complications, it is reserved for patients with DM1 who meet a certain criteria. Concurrent pancreatic and kidney or pancreatic after kidney transplantation are utilized for uremic patients with end-stage renal disease on dialysis or requiring dialysis within 6 months. Pancreatic transplant alone is reserved for patients with DM1 with serious, progressive complications with poor quality of life. Examples include patients with a history of frequent hypoglycemia with unawareness, marked hyperglycemia/multiple episodes of diabetic ketoacidosis, incapacitating clinical distress from exogenous insulin therapy, or continuous failure of insulin-based management to prevent acute complications. Absolute contraindications include age greater than 65, major cardiovascular risk factors, incurable malignancy, active sepsis, peptic ulcer disease, immune suppression, a major psychiatric history which could lead to medication non-adherence, and inability to withstand surgery [165].

Successful transplantation have shown to restore glucose counter regulation [166, 167], induce normalization of HbA1c, improve lipid profiles, and gradually reverse the long-term complications of diabetes [168]. Pancreatic transplant was shown to reduce cardiac risk factors such as decreased total and low-density lipoprotein levels and reduced systolic and diastolic blood pressures, therefore improved cardiac health in patients with DM1 [169]. After 5 years of euglycemia, pancreatic transplantation has been shown to reverse the lesions seen in diabetic nephropathy [170]. In terms of peripheral neuropathy, restoration of motor and sensory function was seen after 12 months of euglycemia post-pancreatic transplant [171].

Although improvements in surgical techniques and immunosuppressive agents have improved patient and graft survival rates [172], there are some downsides and complications of transplantation. In terms of surgical complications, wound infections, graft thrombosis, acute rejection, and anastomotic leaks have been reported [173]. From 2016 to 2020, within the first 3 months posttransplant, 43% of all deaths were caused by cardiac and cerebrovascular events and 25% by infections. From 3 to 12 months posttransplant, infections accounted for 24% and cardiac and cerebrovascular causes were 23% [162]. Although there have been improvements in outcome and survival rate, there has been a decline in the number of pancreatic transplants over the past decade. This is attributed to improved insulin delivery systems, inadequate promotion of positive outcomes of pancreas transplantation by health care providers, insurance coverage, and research initiative shifts to studying islet cell transplantation [174]. Islet transplantation offers a much less inversive alternative to pancreatic transplantation [175].

In June 2023, the FDA Center for Biologics Evaluation and Research approved the first cellular therapy for DM1, called Lantidra [176]. Lantidra (donislecel), developed by the startup company CellTrans, has been approved for adults with DM1 who are unable to reach target glycated hemoglobin levels in the setting of recurrent severe hypoglycemia. The technology uses allogeneic pancreatic islet beta cells transplanted into the recipient's liver via infusion into the hepatic portal vein with the hopes of the donor cells to produce enough insulin so that the recipient no longer needs to take exogenous insulin. The clinical trials show promise; at 1 year, 21 of 30 study participants no longer required insulin, 11 of 30 study participants did not require insulin for between 1 and 5 years, and 10 of 30 study participants did not require insulin for more than 5 years [177]. Although the most common side effects include nausea, fatigue, anemia, abdominal pain, and diarrhea, the most serious drawback is the need to be on immunosuppressive agents to maintain islet cell viability [176]. Another drawback to islet transplantation is the need for multiple donors to provide enough islet cells to achieve insulin dependence [178].

Conclusion

The evolution of insulin delivery systems and the technological advancements we have today has changed the survival trajectory and quality of life of patients with DM1 and DM2 [179]. Survival trajectory of patients with diabetes can be attributed to many factors, such as improvements in blood glucose management, new developments in medications, close follow-up with health care providers, and technological advancements in insulin delivery methods. Although these advancements have led to improved outcomes, it has come with an increase in health care costs and expenditures. Diabetes is the most expensive chronic condition in the United States in which approximately \$1 in every \$4 in US health care costs is spent on caring for people with diabetes [180]. Depending on the method for insulin delivery, raw materials needed to properly manage diabetes can include handheld glucometers, continuous glucose monitors, insulin pumps, insulin, lancet devices, blood glucose test strips, alcohol prep pads, syringes, insulin pens, infusion sets, and many others. A study conducted in 2017 estimated the total economic cost of diabetes in the United States to be $327 USD, of which $237 billion USD secondary to direct medical costs and another $90 billion to indirect medical costs (such as reduced productivity) [180]. The largest contributor of cost is the use of prescription medications, estimated to be $71.2 billion USD annually. A diabetic spends approximately $16,750 USD per year on medical expenditures, which is 2.3 times higher than individuals without the diagnosis of diabetes [180]. With the exponential prevalence of diabetes, trends health care insurance policies, and technological advancements, the economic burden is projected to grow exponentially. Between 2012 and 2017, when adjusted for inflation, it was estimated that the direct medical costs increased by 26% [180]. In a study conducted in 2018, it was estimated that the mean out-of-pocket spending for insulin, diabetes-related supplies, and other health care services for privately insured DM1 persons was $2500 USD annually [181]. On average, an insulin pump costs about $6000 USD and additional supplies (such as infusion sets) can cost between $3000 and $6000 USD annually [182].

Given US stakeholder's involvement in the price of insulin, prices have been exponentially increasing, forcing many insulin-dependent diabetics to ration insulin supply, thus underdosing, leading to worsened clinical outcomes (poor glycemic control, high incidence of diabetic ketoacidosis, and death) [183]. Studies have shown one in four Americans use less insulin than prescribed by their health care professionals secondary to the cost of insulin [60, 184, 185]. The list price of insulin increased by 262% from 2007 to 2018 [186]. The Inflation Reduction Act capped out-of-pocket costs of insulin products at $35 per month for people with Medicare Part D plans (effective January 1, 2023) and Medicare Part B (effective July 1, 2023). Senator John Kennedy and Raphael Warnock introduced the bipartisan Affordable Insulin Now Act of 2023 in March, 2023. The purpose of this bill is to cap the price of insulin for all patients, regardless if insured or uninsured, at $35 for a 30-day supply. Many large insulin manufacturers, including Eli Lily, Novo Nordisk, and Sanofi, have made initiatives of cutting the price of many of their insulins and capping insulin prices to a maximum of $35 per month for insured persons [187–189]. Eli Lilly has provided easy-to-download savings cards that provide a $35 max out-of-pocket monthly cost for people who are uninsured [188].

The evolution of insulin delivery systems has led to extensive improvements in quality of life and longevity of diabetics. Although cost limiting, legislation is currently underway to increase access to diabetes supplies. The desire to develop products to mirror in vivo insulin secretion has led to advancements such as ultra-rapid-acting insulin, insulin pump therapies, and continuous glucose monitors. Understanding the barriers to patient acceptance of insulin usage had led to the creation of noninvasive modes of delivery, such as injection ports, pulmonary, buccal, and oral route. The integration of insulin pump and CGM data has led to immense improvements in outcomes. User-friendly insulin pumps with less advanced capabilities have allowed patients with DM2 to equally benefit from technological advancements without compromising standards of care. The most recent innovative developments in diabetes care, such as automated insulin delivery systems, the bionic pancreas, and cellular therapies, have proven the transformative and expansive nature of the future of diabetes care, with the main objective to improve management to reduce the complication burden of those affected by diabetes. When choosing which strategy to implement, it is important to recognize each insulin delivery system's advantages and disadvantages along with the understanding of new technological advancements and how the system aligns with each individual patient's circumstances, preferences, and needs.

References

1. Tandon N, Kalra S, Balhara YPS, et al. Forum for injection technique and therapy expert recommendations, India: the Indian recommendations for best practice in insulin injection technique, 2017. Indian J Endocrinol Metab. 2017;21(4):600–17. https://doi.org/10.4103/ijem.IJEM_97_17.
2. Nathan DM, Cleary PA, Backlund JY, et al. Intensive diabetes treatment and cardiovascular disease in patients with type 1 diabetes. N Engl J Med. 2005;353(25):2643–53. https://doi.org/10.1056/NEJMoa052187.
3. Diabetes Control and Complications Trial Research Group, Nathan DM, Genuth S, et al. The effect of intensive treatment of diabetes on the development and progression of long-term complications in insulin-dependent diabetes mellitus. N Engl J Med. 1993;329(14):977–86. https://doi.org/10.1056/NEJM199309303291401.
4. Epidemiology of Diabetes Interventions and Complications (EDIC) Research Group, Epidemiology of Diabetes Interventions and Complications (EDIC). Design, implementation, and preliminary results of a long-term follow-up of the Diabetes Control and Complications Trial cohort. Diabetes Care. 1999;22(1):99–111. https://doi.org/10.2337/diacare.22.1.99.
5. El Sayed NA, Aleppo G, Aroda VR, et al. Diabetes technology: standards of care in diabetes-2023. Diabetes Care. 2023;46(Suppl. 1):S111–27. https://doi.org/10.2337/dc23-S007.
6. Our Company BD. www.bd.com. 2023. Accessed August 6, 2023. https://www.bd.com/en-us/about-bd/our-company#accordion-039e4be049-item-41ea369933.
7. Fry A. Insulin delivery device technology 2012: where are we after 90 years? J Diabetes Sci Technol. 2012;6(4):947–53. https://doi.org/10.1177/193229681200600428.
8. Heinemann L, Nguyen T, Bailey TS, et al. Needle technology for insulin administration: a century of innovation. J Diabetes Sci Technol. 2023;17(2):449–57. https://doi.org/10.1177/19322968211059564.
9. Shaw KF, Valdez CA. Development and implementation of a U-500 regular insulin program in a Federally Qualified Health Center. Clin Diabetes. 2017;35(3):162–7. https://doi.org/10.2337/cd16-0057.
10. Gibney MA, Arce CH, Byron KJ, Hirsch LJ. Skin and subcutaneous adipose layer thickness in adults with diabetes at sites used for insulin injections: implications for needle length recommendations. Curr Med Res Opin. 2010;26(6):1519–30.
11. Aronson R, Gibney MA, Oza K, Bérubé J, Kassler-Taub K, Hirsch L. Insulin pen needles: effects of extra-thin wall needle technology on preference, confidence, and other patient ratings. Clin Ther. 2013;35(7):923–933.e4. https://doi.org/10.1016/j.clinthera.2013.05.020.
12. Pearson TL. Practical aspects of insulin pen devices. J Diabetes Sci Technol. 2010;4(3):522–31.
13. Fu AZ, Qiu Y, Radican L. Impact of fear of insulin or fear of injection on treatment outcomes of patients with diabetes. Curr Med Res Opin. 2009;25:1413–20.

14. Graff MR, McClanahan MA. Assessment by patients with diabetes mellitus of two insulin pen delivery systems versus a vial and syringe. Clin Ther. 1998;20(3):486–96.
15. Brunton S. Insulin delivery systems: reducing barriers to insulin therapy and advancing diabetes mellitus treatment. Am J Med. 2008;121(Suppl. 6):S35–41. https://doi.org/10.1016/j.amjmed.2008.03.025.
16. Mollema ED, Snoek FJ, Heine RJ, van der Ploeg HM. Phobia of self-injecting and self-testing in insulin-treated diabetes patients: opportunities for screening. Diabet Med. 2001;18(8):671–4.
17. Dunne T, Whitaker D. Prefilled insulin syringes. Anaesthesia. 2016;71:349–50. https://doi.org/10.1111/anae.13389.
18. Asakura T. Comparison of clinically relevant technical attributes of five insulin injection pens. J Diabetes Sci Technol. 2011;5(5):1203–9. https://doi.org/10.1177/193229681100500527.
19. Rex J, Jensen KH, Lawton SA. A review of 20 years' experience with the NovoPen family of insulin injection devices. Clin Drug Investig. 2006;26(7):367–401. https://doi.org/10.2165/00044011-200626070-00001.
20. Ignaut DA, Venekamp WJ. HumaPen Memoir: a novel insulin injecting pen with a dose-memory feature. Expert Rev Med Devices. 2007;4:793–802.
21. Pfützner A, Schipper C, Niemeyer M, et al. Comparison of patient preference for two insulin injection pen devices in relation to patient dexterity skills. J Diabetes Sci Technol. 2012;6(4):910–6. https://doi.org/10.1177/193229681200600423.
22. Allstar-Sanofi India. Home page—Sanofi India. 2023. Accessed September 10, 2023. https://www.sanofi.in/en/allstar.
23. InPen Meet the inpen TM system—an insulin pen, but smarter. 2023. Retrieved from https://www.medtronicdiabetes.com/products/inpen-smart-insulin-pen-system.
24. Saint S. PR Newswire. Companion Medical Announces U.S. Commercial Launch of Smart Insulin Pen System; 2017. Available at: https://www.prnewswire.com/news-releases/companion-medical-announces-us-commercial-launch-of-smart-insulin-pen-system-300571413.html (Accessed 8.31.2023).
25. Eli Lilly. Eli Lilly is focusing on its successful drug portfolio and is halting its ambition to enter insulin pump business. Ypsomed remains committed to its US YpsoPump ambitions with a new partner. www.ypsomed.com. 2022. Published December 9, 2022. Accessed September 25, 2023. https://www.ypsomed.com/en/media/details/eli-lilly-is-focusing-on-its-successful-drug-portfolio.html.
26. Masierek M, Nabrdalik K, Janota O, Kwiendacz H, Macherski M, Gumprecht J. The review of insulin pens-past, present, and look to the future. Front Endocrinol (Lausanne). 2022;13:827484. https://doi.org/10.3389/fendo.2022.827484.
27. Hyllested-Winge J, Sparre T, Pedersen LK. NovoPen Echo(®) insulin delivery device. Med Devices (Auckl). 2016;9:11–8. https://doi.org/10.2147/MDER.S59229.
28. Access & Affordability. www.novonordisk-us.com. 2023. Accessed September 1, 2023. https://www.novonordisk-us.com/patient-help/access-and-affordability.html.
29. Adolfsson P, Veijola R, Huot C, Hansen HD, Lademann JB, Phillip M. Safety and patient perception of an insulin pen with simple memory function for children and adolescents with type 1 diabetes—the REMIND study. Curr Med Res Opin. 2012;28(9):1455–63. https://doi.org/10.1185/03007995.2012.698258.
30. Asakura T, Jensen KH. Comparison of intuitiveness, ease of use, and preference in two insulin pens. J Diabetes Sci Technol. 2009;3(2):312–9. https://doi.org/10.1177/193229680900300212.
31. Cerna L, Maresova P. Patients' attitudes to the use of modern technologies in the treatment of diabetes. Patient Prefer Adherence. 2016;10:1869–79. https://doi.org/10.2147/PPA.S118040.
32. Olsen BS, Lilleøre SK, Korsholm CN, Kracht T. Novopen Echo® for the delivery of insulin: a comparison of usability, functionality and preference among pediatric subjects, their parents, and health care professionals. J Diabetes Sci Technol. 2010;4(6):1468–75. https://doi.org/10.1177/193229681000400622.

33. Klausmann G, Hramiak I, Qvist M, Mikkelsen KH, Guo X. Evaluation of preference for a novel durable insulin pen with memory function among patients with diabetes and health care professionals. Patient Prefer Adherence. 2013;7:285–92. https://doi.org/10.2147/PPA.S41929.
34. Hyllested-Winge J, Jensen KH, Rex J. A review of 25 years' experience with the NovoPen family of insulin pens in the management of diabetes mellitus. Clin Drug Investig. 2010;30(10):643–74.
35. Pfutzner A, Asakura T, Sommavilla B, Lee W. Insulin delivery with FlexPen: dose accuracy, patient preference and adherence. Expert Opin Drug Deliv. 2008;5(8):915–25.
36. Lombardo F, Salzano G, Messina MF, De Luca F. Compliance and administration methods in management of type 1 diabetes. Acta Biomed. 2005;76(Suppl. 3):66–9.
37. Saha S. Smart insulin pens market to grow at a CAGR of 17.9% through 2027: future market insights. 2018. Available from globenewswire.com/news-release/2018/07/16/1537595/0/en/Smart-Insulin-Pens-Market-to-Grow-at-a-CAGR-of-17-9-through-2027-Future-Market-Insights.html. Accessed 25 July 2018.
38. Karter AJ, Subramanian U, Saha C, et al. Barriers to insulin initiation: the translating research into action for diabetes insulin starts project. Diabetes Care. 2010;33(4):733–5. https://doi.org/10.2337/dc09-1184.
39. Stinson FS, Dawson DA, Patricia Chou S, et al. The epidemiology of DSM-IV specific phobia in the USA: results from the National Epidemiologic Survey on Alcohol and Related Conditions. Psychol Med. 2007;37(7):1047–59. https://doi.org/10.1017/S0033291707000086.
40. Medtronic i-Port Advance injection Port. n.d.. Available from http://www.medtronicdiabetes.com/products/i-port-advance.
41. Khan AM, Alswat KA. Benefits of using the i-Port system on insulin-treated patients. Diabetes Spectr. 2019;32(1):30–5. https://doi.org/10.2337/ds18-0015.
42. Medtronic presents U.S. Pivotal Trial Data for MiniMedTM 780G Advanced Hybrid closed loop system with automated correction bolus feature. Medtronic News. 2023. Accessed September 21, 2023. https://news.medtronic.com/2020-06-12-Medtronic-Presents-U-S-Pivotal-Trial-Data-for-MiniMed-TM-780G-Advanced-Hybrid-Closed-Loop-System-with-Automated-Correction-Bolus-Feature.
43. Kadish AH. A servomechanism for blood sugar control. Biomed Sci Instrum. 1963;1:171–6.
44. Cobelli C, Renard E, Kovatchev B. Artificial pancreas: past, present, future. Diabetes. 2011;60(11):2672–82. https://doi.org/10.2337/db11-0654.
45. Kerr D, Morton J, Whately-Smith C, Everett J, Begley JP. Laboratory-based non-clinical comparison of occlusion rates using three rapid-acting insulin analogs in continuous subcutaneous insulin infusion catheters using low flow rates. J Diabetes Sci Technol. 2008;2(3):450–5. https://doi.org/10.1177/193229680800200314.
46. Insulin pump market size, share & covid-19 impact analysis, by product type (pumps [tethered pumps, patch pumps, and others] and consumables), by disease indication (type 1 diabetes and type 2 diabetes), by Distribution Channel (Hospital Pharmacy and Retail & Online Pharmacy), and Regional Forecast, 2023-2030. Insulin Pump Market Size, Share, Growth | Global Report. 2030. Accessed August 25, 2023. https://www.fortunebusinessinsights.com/insulin-pump-market-102735.
47. Buse JB, Kudva YC, Battelino T, Davis SN, Shin J, Welsh JB. Effects of sensor-augmented pump therapy on glycemic variability in well-controlled type 1 diabetes in the STAR 3 study. Diabetes Technol Ther. 2012;14(7):644–7. https://doi.org/10.1089/dia.2011.0294.
48. Steineck I, Ranjan A, Nørgaard K, Schmidt S. Sensor-augmented insulin pumps and hypoglycemia prevention in type 1 diabetes. J Diabetes Sci Technol. 2017;11(1):50–8. https://doi.org/10.1177/1932296816672689.
49. Garg S, Brazg RL, Bailey TS, et al. Reduction in duration of hypoglycemia by automatic suspension of insulin delivery: the in-clinic ASPIRE study. Diabetes Technol Ther. 2012;14(3):205–9.

50. Ly TT, Nicholas JA, Retterath A, Lim EM, Davis EA, Jones TW. Effect of sensor-augmented insulin pump therapy and automated insulin suspension vs standard insulin pump therapy on hypoglycemia in patients with type 1 diabetes: a randomized clinical trial. JAMA. 2013;310(12):1240–7.
51. Choudhary P, Shin J, Wang Y, et al. Insulin pump therapy with automated insulin suspension in response to hypoglycemia: reduction in nocturnal hypoglycemia in those at greatest risk. Diabetes Care. 2011;34(9):2023–5.
52. Brazg RL, Bailey TS, Garg S, et al. The ASPIRE study: design and methods of an in-clinic crossover trial on the efficacy of automatic insulin pump suspension in exercise-induced hypoglycemia. J Diabetes Sci Technol. 2011;5(6):1466–71. https://doi.org/10.1177/193229681100500621.
53. Cappon G, Vettoretti M, Sparacino G, Facchinetti A. Continuous glucose monitoring sensors for diabetes management: a review of technologies and applications. Diabetes Metab J. 2019;43(4):383–97. https://doi.org/10.4093/dmj.2019.0121.
54. Juvenile Diabetes Research Foundation Continuous Glucose Monitoring Study Group, Tamborlane WV, Beck RW, et al. Continuous glucose monitoring and intensive treatment of type 1 diabetes. N Engl J Med. 2008;359(14):1464–76. https://doi.org/10.1056/NEJMoa0805017.
55. Beck RW, Riddlesworth T, Ruedy K, et al. Effect of continuous glucose monitoring on glycemic control in adults with type 1 diabetes using insulin injections: the DIAMOND randomized clinical trial. JAMA. 2017;317(4):371–8. https://doi.org/10.1001/jama.2016.19975.
56. Pratley RE, Kanapka LG, Rickels MR, et al. Effect of continuous glucose monitoring on hypoglycemia in older adults with type 1 diabetes: a randomized clinical trial. JAMA. 2020;323(23):2397–406. https://doi.org/10.1001/jama.2020.6928.
57. Heinemann L, Freckmann G, Ehrmann D, et al. Real-time continuous glucose monitoring in adults with type 1 diabetes and impaired hypoglycaemia awareness or severe hypoglycaemia treated with multiple daily insulin injections (HypoDE): a multicentre, randomised controlled trial. Lancet. 2018;391(10128):1367–77. https://doi.org/10.1016/S0140-6736(18)30297-6.
58. Tumminia A, Crimi S, Sciacca L, et al. Efficacy of real-time continuous glucose monitoring on glycaemic control and glucose variability in type 1 diabetic patients treated with either insulin pumps or multiple insulin injection therapy: a randomized controlled crossover trial. Diabetes Metab Res Rev. 2015;31(1):61–8. https://doi.org/10.1002/dmrr.2557.
59. Aleppo G, Beck RW, Bailey R, et al. The effect of discontinuing continuous glucose monitoring in adults with type 2 diabetes treated with basal insulin. Diabetes Care. 2021;44(12):2729–37. https://doi.org/10.2337/dc21-1304.
60. Luo J, Gellad WF. Origins of the crisis in insulin affordability and practical advice for clinicians on using human insulin. Curr Diab Rep. 2020;20(1):2. https://doi.org/10.1007/s11892-020-1286-3.
61. Herman A, de Montjoye L, Baeck M. Adverse cutaneous reaction to diabetic glucose sensors and insulin pumps: irritant contact dermatitis or allergic contact dermatitis? Contact Dermatitis. 2020;83(1):25–30. https://doi.org/10.1111/cod.13529.
62. Basu A, Slama MQ, Nicholson WT, et al. Continuous glucose monitor interference with commonly prescribed medications: a pilot study. J Diabetes Sci Technol. 2017;11(5):936–41. https://doi.org/10.1177/1932296817697329.
63. Calhoun P, Johnson TK, Hughes J, Price D, Balo AK. Resistance to acetaminophen interference in a novel continuous glucose monitoring system. J Diabetes Sci Technol. 2018;12(2):393–6. https://doi.org/10.1177/1932296818755797.
64. Szmuilowicz ED, Aleppo G. Interferent effect of hydroxyurea on continuous glucose monitoring. Diabetes Care. 2021;44(5):e89–90. https://doi.org/10.2337/dc20-3114.
65. Lewis DM. Do-it-yourself artificial pancreas system and the OpenAPS movement. Endocrinol Metab Clin North Am. 2020;49(1):203–13. https://doi.org/10.1016/j.ecl.2019.10.005.
66. Weaver KW, Hirsch IB. The hybrid closed-loop system: evolution and practical applications. Diabetes Technol Ther. 2018;20:S216–23.

67. Brown SA, Kovatchev BP, Raghinaru D, et al. Six-month randomized, multicenter trial of closed-loop control in type 1 diabetes. N Engl J Med. 2019;381(18):1707–17. https://doi.org/10.1056/NEJMoa1907863.
68. Lal RA, Basina M, Maahs DM, Hood K, Buckingham B, Wilson DM. One year clinical experience of the first commercial hybrid closed-loop system. Diabetes Care. 2019;42(12):2190–6. https://doi.org/10.2337/dc19-0855.
69. Kovatchev B, Anderson SM, Raghinaru D, et al. Randomized controlled trial of mobile closed-loop control [published correction appears in Diabetes Care. 2020;43(6):1366]. Diabetes Care. 2020;43(3):607–15. https://doi.org/10.2337/dc19-1310.
70. Sherr JL, Cengiz E, Palerm CC, et al. Reduced hypoglycemia and increased time in target using closed-loop insulin delivery during nights with or without antecedent afternoon exercise in type 1 diabetes. Diabetes Care. 2013;36(10):2909–14. https://doi.org/10.2337/dc13-0010.
71. Barnard KD, Wysocki T, Allen JM, et al. Closing the loop overnight at home setting: psychosocial impact for adolescents with type 1 diabetes and their parents. BMJ Open Diabetes Res Care. 2014;2(1):e000025. https://doi.org/10.1136/bmjdrc-2014-000025.
72. Carlson AL, Sherr JL, Shulman DI, et al. Safety and glycemic outcomes during the MiniMed™ advanced hybrid closed-loop system pivotal trial in adolescents and adults with type 1 diabetes. Diabetes Technol Ther. 2022;24(3):178–89. https://doi.org/10.1089/dia.2021.0319.
73. Commissioner of the FDA authorizes first interoperable insulin pump intended to allow patients to customize treatment through their individual diabetes management devices. FDA. Published February 14, 2019. https://www.fda.gov/news-events/press-announcements/fda-authorizes-first-interoperable-insulin-pump-intended-allow-patients-customize-treatment-through.
74. YpsoPump with mylife Loop—mylife Diabetescare—International. 2023. www.mylife--diabetescare.com. Accessed September 25, 2023. https://www.mylife-diabetescare.com/en/mylife-loop.html.
75. Briskin A. diaTribe | making sense of diabetes. Diatribe.org. Published January 26, 2023. Accessed September 22, 2023. https://diatribe.org/.
76. Taylor NP. Embecta joins Tidepool to develop insulin pump, raises Q2 growth outlook. MedTech Dive. Published May 15, 2023. https://www.medtechdive.com/news/embecta-EMBC-tidepool-insulin-pump-earnings/650238/.
77. Innovation Milestones | Medtronic Diabetes. Medtronicdiabetes.com. Published 2018. Accessed September 1, 2023. https://www.medtronicdiabetes.com/about-medtronic-innovation/milestone-timeline.
78. Zhang G, Cohen O, Chattaraj S. Development of the extended infusion set and its mechanism of action [published online ahead of print, 2022 Jul 25]. J Diabetes Sci Technol. 2022:19322968221112120. https://doi.org/10.1177/19322968221112120.
79. Tandem Mobi, World's smallest durable insulin delivery system, receives FDA clearance | tandem diabetes care. Tandem Diabetes Care. Published 2023. https://investor.tandemdiabetes.com/news-releases/news-release-details/tandem-mobi-worlds-smallest-durable-insulin-delivery-system.
80. Klonoff DC, Ho CN, Ayers A, Abdel-Malek A. FDA Interoperability designation-creating options for people with diabetes and pump companies: regulatory, technological, and commercial perspectives. J Diabetes Sci Technol. Published online September 10, 2024. https://doi.org/10.1177/19322968241271304.
81. Retnakaran R, Hochman J, DeVries JH, et al. Continuous subcutaneous insulin infusion versus multiple daily injections: the impact of baseline A1c. Diabetes Care. 2004;27(11):2590–6. https://doi.org/10.2337/diacare.27.11.2590.
82. Weissberg-Benchell J, Antisdel-Lomaglio J, Seshadri R. Insulin pump therapy: a meta-analysis. Diabetes Care. 2003;26(4):1079–87. https://doi.org/10.2337/diacare.26.4.1079.

83. Pickup JC, Reznik Y, Sutton AJ. Glycemic control during continuous subcutaneous insulin infusion versus multiple daily insulin injections in type 2 diabetes: individual patient data meta-analysis and meta-regression of randomized controlled trials. Diabetes Care. 2017;40(5):715–22. https://doi.org/10.2337/dc16-2201.
84. Maiorino MI, Bellastella G, Casciano O, et al. The effects of subcutaneous insulin infusion versus multiple insulin injections on glucose variability in young adults with type 1 diabetes: the 2-year follow-up of the observational METRO study. Diabetes Technol Ther. 2018;20(2):117–26. https://doi.org/10.1089/dia.2017.0334.
85. Misso ML, Egberts KJ, Page M, O'Connor D, Shaw J. Continuous subcutaneous insulin infusion (CSII) versus multiple insulin injections for type 1 diabetes mellitus. Cochrane Database Syst Rev. 2010;(1):CD005103. https://doi.org/10.1002/14651858.CD005103.pub2.
86. American Diabetes Association Professional Practice Committee. Diabetes technology: standards of medical care in diabetes—2022. Diabetes Care. 2022;45(Suppl. 1):S97–S112. https://doi.org/10.2337/dc22-S007.
87. Bruttomesso D, Costa S, Baritussio A. Continuous subcutaneous insulin infusion (CSII) 30 years later: still the best option for insulin therapy. Diabetes Metab Res Rev. 2009;25(2):99–111. https://doi.org/10.1002/dmrr.931.
88. Foster NC, Beck RW, Miller KM, et al. State of type 1 diabetes management and outcomes from the T1D exchange in 2016–2018. Diabetes Technol Ther. 2019;21(2):66–72. https://doi.org/10.1089/dia.2018.0384.
89. Lin MH, Connor CG, Ruedy KJ, et al. Race, socioeconomic status, and treatment center are associated with insulin pump therapy in youth in the first year following diagnosis of type 1 diabetes. Diabetes Technol Ther. 2013;15(11):929–34. https://doi.org/10.1089/dia.2013.0132.
90. Willi SM, Miller KM, DiMeglio LA, et al. Racial-ethnic disparities in management and outcomes among children with type 1 diabetes. Pediatrics. 2015;135(3):424–34. https://doi.org/10.1542/peds.2014-1774.
91. Agarwal S, Simmonds I, Myers AK. The Use of diabetes technology to address inequity in health outcomes: limitations and opportunities. Curr Diab Rep. 2022;22(7):275–81. https://doi.org/10.1007/s11892-022-01470-3.
92. Sherr JL, Tauschmann M, Battelino T, et al. ISPAD clinical practice consensus guidelines 2018: diabetes technologies. Pediatr Diabetes. 2018;19(Suppl. 27):302–25. https://doi.org/10.1111/pedi.12731.
93. O'Connell MA, Donath S, O'Neal DN, et al. Glycaemic impact of patient-led use of sensor-guided pump therapy in type 1 diabetes: a randomised controlled trial. Diabetologia. 2009;52(7):1250–7. https://doi.org/10.1007/s00125-009-1365-0.
94. Reznik Y, Cohen O. Insulin pump for type 2 diabetes: use and misuse of continuous subcutaneous insulin infusion in type 2 diabetes. Diabetes Care. 2013;36(Suppl. 2):S219–25. https://doi.org/10.2337/dcS13-2027.
95. Vigersky RA, Huang S, Cordero TL, et al. Improved HbA1c, total daily insulin dose, and treatment satisfaction with insulin pump therapy compared to multiple daily insulin injections in patients with type 2 diabetes irrespective of baseline c-peptide levels. Endocr Pract. 2018;24(5):446–52. https://doi.org/10.4158/EP-2017-0234.
96. Aronson R, Reznik Y, Conget I, et al. Sustained efficacy of insulin pump therapy compared with multiple daily injections in type 2 diabetes: 12-month data from the OpT2mise randomized trial. Diabetes Obes Metab. 2016;18(5):500–7. https://doi.org/10.1111/dom.12642.
97. Edelman SV, Bode BW, Bailey TS, et al. Insulin pump therapy in patients with type 2 diabetes safely improved glycemic control using a simple insulin dosing regimen. Diabetes Technol Ther. 2010;12(8):627–33. https://doi.org/10.1089/dia.2010.0034.
98. Freckmann G, Buck S, Waldenmaier D, et al. Insulin pump therapy for patients with type 2 diabetes mellitus: evidence, current barriers, and new technologies [published correction appears in J Diabetes Sci Technol. 2021 Jun 16;:19322968211027984]. J Diabetes Sci Technol. 2021;15(4):901–15. https://doi.org/10.1177/1932296820928100.

99. King AB, Clark D, Wolfe GS. The number of basal rates required to achieve near-normal basal glucose control in pump-treated type 2 diabetes. Diabetes Technol Ther. 2012;14(10):900–3. https://doi.org/10.1089/dia.2012.0104.
100. Hermanns N, Lilly LC, Mader JK, et al. Novel simple insulin delivery device reduces barriers to insulin therapy in type 2 diabetes: results from a pilot study. J Diabetes Sci Technol. 2015;9(3):581–7. https://doi.org/10.1177/1932296815570709.
101. Fill, Wear & Go with V-Go. V-Go. 2023. Accessed August 2, 2023. https://www.go-vgo.com/.
102. Lilly LC, Mader JK, Warner J. Developing a simple 3-day insulin delivery device to meet the needs of people with type 2 diabetes. J Diabetes Sci Technol. 2019;13(1):11–9. https://doi.org/10.1177/1932296818807223.
103. Home | Wearable Insulin Patch | Injection-Free. CeQur Simplicity. 2023. Accessed August 2, 2023. https://myceqursimplicity.com/.
104. Insulet. Insulet Announces FDA Clearance of Omnipod GOTM, a First-of-its-Kind Basal-Only Insulin Pod, Further Simplifying Life for People with Type 2 Diabetes. investors.insulet.com. 2023. Published April 25, 2023. Accessed August 25, 2023. https://investors.insulet.com/news/news-details/2023/Insulet-Announces-FDA-Clearance-of-Omnipod-GO-a-First-of-its-Kind-Basal-Only-Insulin-Pod-Further-Simplifying-Life-for-People-with-Type-2-Diabetes/default.aspx.
105. Bionic Pancreas Research Group, Russell SJ, Beck RW, et al. Multicenter, randomized trial of a bionic pancreas in type 1 diabetes. N Engl J Med. 2022;387(13):1161–72. https://doi.org/10.1056/NEJMoa2205225.
106. HOME. Beta Bionics. 2023. Accessed September 20, 2023. https://www.betabionics.com/.
107. Hunt LM, Valenzuela MA, Pugh JA. NIDDM patients' fears and hopes about insulin therapy. The basis of patient reluctance. Diabetes Care. 1997;20(3):292–8. https://doi.org/10.2337/diacare.20.3.292.
108. Al Hayek AA, Robert AA, Babli S, Almonea K, Al Dawish MA. Fear of self-injecting and self-testing and the related risk factors in adolescents with type 1 diabetes: a cross sectional study. Diabetes Ther. 2017;8(1):75–83. https://doi.org/10.1007/s13300-016-0221-8.
109. Guo L, Xiao X, Sun X, Qi C. Comparison of jet injector and insulin pen in controlling plasma glucose and insulin concentrations in type 2 diabetic patients. Medicine (Baltimore). 2017;96(1):e5482. https://doi.org/10.1097/MD.0000000000005482.
110. Mitragotri S. Current status and future prospects of needle-free liquid jet injectors. Nat Rev Drug Discov. 2006;5(7):543–8. https://doi.org/10.1038/nrd2076.
111. Malone JI, Lowitt S, Grove NP, Shah SC. Comparison of insulin levels after injection by jet stream and disposable insulin syringe. Diabetes Care. 1986;9(6):637–40. https://doi.org/10.2337/diacare.9.6.637.
112. Reutens AT, Balkau B, Cohen N. A pilot study to examine the tolerability and device preference in type 1 diabetes of insulin aspart administered by InsuJet compared with subcutaneous injection. Diabetes Technol Ther. 2014;16(4):235–40. https://doi.org/10.1089/dia.2013.0250.
113. Engwerda EE, Tack CJ, de Galan BE. Needle-free jet injection of rapid-acting insulin improves early postprandial glucose control in patients with diabetes. Diabetes Care. 2013;36(11):3436–41. https://doi.org/10.2337/dc13-0492.
114. de Wit HM, Engwerda EE, Tack CJ, de Galan BE. Insulin administered by needle-free jet injection corrects marked hyperglycaemia faster in overweight or obese patients with diabetes. Diabetes Obes Metab. 2015;17(11):1093–9. https://doi.org/10.1111/dom.12550.
115. Ohtake S, Kolhe P. Conventional and nontraditional delivery methods and routes of vaccine administration. In: Practical aspects of vaccine development. Academic Press, an imprint of Elsevier; 2022. p. 329–55.
116. Sonoki K, Yoshinari M, Iwase M, et al. Regurgitation of blood into insulin cartridges in the pen-like injectors. Diabetes Care. 2001;24(3):603–4. https://doi.org/10.2337/diacare.24.3.603.
117. InsuJet. InsuJet store—needlle-free insulin jet administration system. InsuJet; 2023. Accessed August 5, 2023. https://www.insujet.com/

118. National Center for Immunization and Respiratory Diseases. General recommendations on immunization—recommendations of the Advisory Committee on Immunization Practices (ACIP) [published correction appears in MMWR Recomm Rep. 2011 Jul 29;60:993]. MMWR Recomm Rep. 2011;60(2):1–64.
119. Kesavadev J, Saboo B, Krishna MB, Krishnan G. Evolution of insulin delivery devices: from syringes, pens, and pumps to DIY artificial pancreas. Diabetes Ther. 2020;11(6):1251–69. https://doi.org/10.1007/s13300-020-00831-z.
120. Bremseth DL, Pass F. Delivery of insulin by jet injection: recent observations. Diabetes Technol Ther. 2001;3(2):225–32. https://doi.org/10.1089/152091501300209598.
121. Houtzagers CM, Visser AP, Berntzen PA, Heine RJ, van der Veen EA. The Medi-Jector II: efficacy and acceptability in insulin-dependent diabetic patients with and without needle phobia. Diabet Med. 1988;5(2):135–8. https://doi.org/10.1111/j.1464-5491.1988.tb00959.x.
122. Rayman G, Walker R, Day JL. Patient experience with a jet injector. Diabet Med. 1989;6(3):274–6. https://doi.org/10.1111/j.1464-5491.1989.tb01160.x.
123. Resman Z, Metelko Z, Skrabalo Z. The application of insulin using the jet injector DG-77. Acta Diabetol Lat. 1985;22(2):119–25. https://doi.org/10.1007/BF02590785.
124. Maberly GF, Wait GA, Kilpatrick JA, et al. Evidence for insulin degradation by muscle and fat tissue in an insulin resistant diabetic patient. Diabetologia. 1982;23(4):333–6. https://doi.org/10.1007/BF00253740.
125. Garcia-Verdugo R, Erbach M, Schnell O. A new optimized percutaneous access system for CIPII. J Diabetes Sci Technol. 2017;11(4):814–21. https://doi.org/10.1177/1932296817694913.
126. van Dijk PR, Logtenberg SJ, Groenier KH, et al. Continuous intraperitoneal insulin infusion in type 1 diabetes: a 6-year post-trial follow-up. BMC Endocr Disord. 2014;14:30. https://doi.org/10.1186/1472-6823-14-30.
127. Rieger C, Kurz K, Mueller-Hoffmann W, Gehr B, Liebl A. New design of a percutaneous port system for continuous intraperitoneal insulin infusion. J Diabetes Sci Technol. 2019;13(6):1158–60. https://doi.org/10.1177/1932296819855425.
128. Dirnena-Fusini I, Åm MK, Fougner AL, Carlsen SM, Christiansen SC. Physiological effects of intraperitoneal versus subcutaneous insulin infusion in patients with diabetes mellitus type 1: a systematic review and meta-analysis. PLoS One. 2021;16(4):e0249611. https://doi.org/10.1371/journal.pone.0249611.
129. van Dijk PR, Logtenberg SJ, Groenier KH, Haveman JW, Kleefstra N, Bilo HJ. Complications of continuous intraperitoneal insulin infusion with an implantable pump. World J Diabetes. 2012;3(8):142–8. https://doi.org/10.4239/wjd.v3.i8.142.
130. Owens DR, Zinman B, Bolli G. Alternative routes of insulin delivery. Diabet Med. 2003;20(11):886–98. https://doi.org/10.1046/j.1464-5491.2003.01076.x.
131. Rave K, Bott S, Heinemann L, et al. Time-action profile of inhaled insulin in comparison with subcutaneously injected insulin lispro and regular human insulin. Diabetes Care. 2005;28(5):1077–82. https://doi.org/10.2337/diacare.28.5.1077.
132. Oleck J, Kassam S, Goldman JD. Commentary: why was inhaled insulin a failure in the market? Diabetes Spectr. 2016;29(3):180–4. https://doi.org/10.2337/diaspect.29.3.180.
133. Bailey Clifford J, Barnett AH. Why is Exubera being withdrawn? BMJ. 2007;335(7630):1156.
134. Heinemann L. The failure of exubera: are we beating a dead horse? J Diabetes Sci Technol. 2008;2(3):518–29. https://doi.org/10.1177/193229680800200325.
135. Klonoff DC. Afrezza inhaled insulin: the fastest-acting FDA-approved insulin on the market has favorable properties. J Diabetes Sci Technol. 2014;8(6):1071–3. https://doi.org/10.1177/1932296814555820.
136. Testa MA, Simonson DC. Satisfaction and quality of life with premeal inhaled versus injected insulin in adolescents and adults with type 1 diabetes. Diabetes Care. 2007;30(6):1399–405. https://doi.org/10.2337/dc06-1497.
137. Afrezza. 2023. https://afrezza.com/wp-content/uploads/2023/02/Medication-Guide-Feb-2023.pdf.

138. Yeh HC, Punjabi NM, Wang NY, et al. Cross-sectional and prospective study of lung function in adults with type 2 diabetes: the Atherosclerosis Risk in Communities (ARIC) study. Diabetes Care. 2008;31(4):741–6. https://doi.org/10.2337/dc07-1464.
139. McGill JB, Peters A, Buse JB, et al. Comprehensive pulmonary safety review of inhaled Technosphere® insulin in patients with diabetes mellitus. Clin Drug Investig. 2020;40(10):973–83. https://doi.org/10.1007/s40261-020-00958-8.
140. Edgerton DS, Moore MC, Winnick JJ, et al. Changes in glucose and fat metabolism in response to the administration of a hepato-preferential insulin analog. Diabetes. 2014;63(11):3946–54. https://doi.org/10.2337/db14-0266.
141. Elsayed AM. Oral delivery of insulin: novel approaches. In: Recent advances in novel drug carrier systems, vol. 281. London, UK: InTech; 2012.
142. Shah RB, Patel M, Maahs DM, Shah VN. Insulin delivery methods: past, present and future. Int J Pharm Investig. 2016;6(1):1–9. https://doi.org/10.4103/2230-973X.176456.
143. Lassmann-Vague V, Raccah D. Alternatives routes of insulin delivery. Diabetes Metab. 2006;32(5 Pt 2):513–22. https://doi.org/10.1016/s1262-3636(06)72804-x.
144. Ziv E, Lior O, Kidron M. Absorption of protein via the intestinal wall. A quantitative model. Biochem Pharmacol. 1987;36(7):1035–9. https://doi.org/10.1016/0006-2952(87)90411-4.
145. Lebovitz HE, Fleming A, Cherrington AD, et al. Efficacy and safety of Tregopil, a novel, ultra-rapid acting oral prandial insulin analog, as part of a basal-bolus regimen in type 2 diabetes: a randomized, active-controlled phase 2/3 study. Expert Opin Pharmacother. 2022;23(16):1855–63. https://doi.org/10.1080/14656566.2022.2141569.
146. Kisel MA, Kulik LN, Tsybovsky IS, et al. Liposomes with phosphatidylethanol as a carrier for oral delivery of insulin: studies in the rat. Int J Pharm. 2001;216(1-2):105–14. https://doi.org/10.1016/s0378-5173(01)00579-8.
147. Kim BY, Jeong JH, Park K, Kim JD. Bioadhesive interaction and hypoglycemic effect of insulin-loaded lectin-microparticle conjugates in oral insulin delivery system. J Control Release. 2005;102(3):525–38. https://doi.org/10.1016/j.jconrel.2004.10.032.
148. Sharma G, Sharma AR, Nam JS, Doss GP, Lee SS, Chakraborty C. Nanoparticle based insulin delivery system: the next generation efficient therapy for Type 1 diabetes. J Nanobiotechnol. 2015;13:74. https://doi.org/10.1186/s12951-015-0136-y.
149. Eldor R, Francis BH, Fleming A, et al. Oral insulin (ORMD-0801) in type 2 diabetes mellitus: a dose-finding 12-week randomized placebo-controlled study. Diabetes Obes Metab. 2023;25(4):943–52. https://doi.org/10.1111/dom.14901.
150. Inc OP. Oramed Announces Top-line Results from Phase 3 Trial of ORMD-0801 for the Treatment of Type 2 Diabetes. www.prnewswire.com. Published January 11, 2023. Accessed September 26, 2023. https://www.prnewswire.com/news-releases/oramed-announces-top-line-results-from-phase-3-trial-of-ormd-0801-for-the-treatment-of-type-2-diabetes-301719709.html#:~:text=The%20ORA%2DD%2D013%2D.
151. Oramed Announces that its Chinese Partner, HTIT, has Successfully Completed a Phase 3 Oral Insulin Clinical Trial and Submitted a Marketing Authorization Application in China. BioSpace. Published May 15, 2023. Accessed September 26, 2023. https://www.biospace.com/article/releases/oramed-announces-that-its-chinese-partner-htit-has-successfully-completed-a-phase-3-oral-insulin-clinical-trial-and-submitted-a-marketing-authorization-application-in-china/.
152. New RRC, Ramanujam S, Chaudhari V, Bogus M, Travers GN, Namjoshi G. Safety and efficacy of an oral insulin (Capsulin) in patients with early-stage type 2 diabetes: a dose-ranging phase 2b study. Diabetes Obes Metab. 2023;25(4):953–60. https://doi.org/10.1111/dom.14922.
153. Rachmiel M, Barash G, Leshem A, Sagi R, Doenyas-barak K, Koren S. OR14-1 Pharmacodynamics, safety, tolerability, and efficacy of oral insulin formulation (Oshadi Icp) among young adults with type 1 diabetes: a summary of clinical studies phases I, Ib, and Ii. J Endocr Soc. 2019;3(Suppl 1):OR14-1. https://doi.org/10.1210/js.2019-OR14-1.

154. Weinstock RS, Bode BW, Garg SK, et al. Reduced hypoglycaemia using liver-targeted insulin in individuals with type 1 diabetes. Diabetes Obes Metab. 2022;24(9):1762–9. https://doi.org/10.1111/dom.14761.
155. Malkov D, Angelo R, Wang HZ, Flanders E, Tang H, Gomez-Orellana I. Oral delivery of insulin with the eligen technology: mechanistic studies. Curr Drug Deliv. 2005;2(2):191–7. https://doi.org/10.2174/1567201053586001.
156. Iyer G, Dyawanapelly S, Jain R, Dandekar P. An overview of oral insulin delivery strategies (OIDS). Int J Biol Macromol. 2022;208:565–85. https://doi.org/10.1016/j.ijbiomac.2022.03.144.
157. Arbit E, Kidron M. Oral insulin delivery in a physiologic context: review. J Diabetes Sci Technol. 2017;11(4):825–32. https://doi.org/10.1177/1932296817691303.
158. Guevara-Aguirre J, Guevara-Aguirre M, Saavedra J, Bernstein G, Rosenbloom AL. Comparison of oral insulin spray and subcutaneous regular insulin at mealtime in type 1 diabetes. Diabetes Technol Ther. 2007;9(4):372–6. https://doi.org/10.1089/dia.2006.0019.
159. Mauer M, Fioretto P. Pancreas transplantation and reversal of diabetic nephropathy lesions. Med Clin North Am. 2013;97(1):109–14. https://doi.org/10.1016/j.mcna.2012.10.009.
160. Kelly WD, Lillehei RC, Merkel FK, Idezuki Y, Goetz FC. Allotransplantation of the pancreas and duodenum along with the kidney in diabetic nephropathy. Surgery. 1967;61(6):827–37.
161. Dholakia S, Oskrochi Y, Easton G, Papalois V. Advances in pancreas transplantation. J R Soc Med. 2016;109(4):141–6. https://doi.org/10.1177/0141076816636369.
162. Gruessner AC, Gruessner RWG. The 2022 International pancreas transplant registry report—a review. Transplant Proc. 2022;54(7):1918–43. https://doi.org/10.1016/j.transproceed.2022.03.059.
163. Margreiter C, Resch T, Oberhuber R, et al. Combined pancreas-kidney transplantation for patients with end-stage nephropathy caused by type-2 diabetes mellitus. Transplantation. 2013;95(8):1030–6. https://doi.org/10.1097/TP.0b013e3182861945.
164. Sampaio MS, Kuo HT, Bunnapradist S. Outcomes of simultaneous pancreas-kidney transplantation in type 2 diabetic recipients. Clin J Am Soc Nephrol. 2011;6(5):1198–206. https://doi.org/10.2215/CJN.06860810.
165. Bahar SG, Devulapally P. Pancreas transplantation. StatPearls Publishing; 2023. Accessed October 4, 2023. https://www.ncbi.nlm.nih.gov/books/NBK562338/?report=reader#_NBK562338_pubdet_
166. Rickels MR, Fuller C, Dalton-Bakes C, et al. Restoration of glucose counterregulation by islet transplantation in long-standing type 1 diabetes. Diabetes. 2015;64(5):1713–8. https://doi.org/10.2337/db14-1620.
167. Robertson RP, Sutherland DE, Seaquist ER, Lanz KJ. Glucagon, catecholamine, and symptom responses to hypoglycemia in living donors of pancreas segments. Diabetes. 2003;52(7):1689–94. https://doi.org/10.2337/diabetes.52.7.1689.
168. Fiorina P, Folli F, Bertuzzi F, et al. Long-term beneficial effect of islet transplantation on diabetic macro-/microangiopathy in type 1 diabetic kidney-transplanted patients. Diabetes Care. 2003;26(4):1129–36. https://doi.org/10.2337/diacare.26.4.1129.
169. Coppelli A, Giannarelli R, Mariotti R, et al. Pancreas transplant alone determines early improvement of cardiovascular risk factors and cardiac function in type 1 diabetic patients. Transplantation. 2003;76(6):974–6. https://doi.org/10.1097/01.TP.0000084202.18999.1D.
170. Fioretto P, Steffes MW, Sutherland DE, Goetz FC, Mauer M. Reversal of lesions of diabetic nephropathy after pancreas transplantation. N Engl J Med. 1998;339(2):69–75. https://doi.org/10.1056/NEJM199807093390202.
171. Kennedy WR, Navarro X, Goetz FC, Sutherland DE, Najarian JS. Effects of pancreatic transplantation on diabetic neuropathy. N Engl J Med. 1990;322(15):1031–7. https://doi.org/10.1056/NEJM199004123221503.
172. Sutherland DE, Gruessner RW, Dunn DL, et al. Lessons learned from more than 1000 pancreas transplants at a single institution. Ann Surg. 2001;233(4):463–501. https://doi.org/10.1097/00000658-200104000-00003.

173. Gruessner AC, Sutherland DE. Pancreas transplant outcomes for United States (US) cases as reported to the United Network for Organ Sharing (UNOS) and the International Pancreas Transplant Registry (IPTR). Clin Transpl. 2008:45–56.
174. Gruessner AC, Gruessner RW. Declining numbers of pancreas transplantations but significant improvements in outcome. Transplant Proc. 2014;46(6):1936–7. https://doi.org/10.1016/j.transproceed.2014.06.045.
175. Rickels MR, Robertson RP. Pancreatic islet transplantation in humans: recent progress and future directions. Endocr Rev. 2019;40(2):631–68. https://doi.org/10.1210/er.2018-00154.
176. Food and Drug Administration (FDA) News Release. FDA approves first cellular therapy to treat patients with type 1 diabetes. Jun 28, 2023. Available at: https://www.fda.gov/news-events/press-announcements/fda-approves-first-cellular-therapy-treat-patients-type-1-diabetes#.
177. Harris E. FDA greenlights first cell therapy for adults with type 1 diabetes. JAMA. 2023;330(5):402. https://doi.org/10.1001/jama.2023.12542.
178. Yang L, Hu ZM, Jiang FX, Wang W. Stem cell therapy for insulin-dependent diabetes: Are we still on the road? World J Stem Cells. 2022;14(7):503–12. https://doi.org/10.4252/wjsc.v14.i7.503.
179. Miller RG, Secrest AM, Sharma RK, Songer TJ, Orchard TJ. Improvements in the life expectancy of type 1 diabetes: the Pittsburgh Epidemiology of Diabetes Complications study cohort. Diabetes. 2012;61(11):2987–92. https://doi.org/10.2337/db11-1625.
180. American Diabetes Association. Economic costs of diabetes in the U.S. in 2017. Diabetes Care. 2018;41(5):917–28. https://doi.org/10.2337/dci18-0007.
181. Chua KP, Lee JM, Conti RM. Out-of-pocket spending for insulin, diabetes-related supplies, and other health care services among privately insured US patients with type 1 diabetes. JAMA Intern Med. 2020;180(7):1012–4. https://doi.org/10.1001/jamainternmed.2020.1308.
182. McAdams BH, Rizvi AA. An overview of insulin pumps and glucose sensors for the generalist. J Clin Med. 2016;5(1):5. https://doi.org/10.3390/jcm5010005.
183. Beran D, Hirsch IB, Yudkin JS. Why are we failing to address the issue of access to insulin? A national and global perspective [published correction appears in diabetes care]. Diabetes Care. 2018;41(6):1125–31. https://doi.org/10.2337/dc17-2123.
184. Herkert D, Vijayakumar P, Luo J, et al. Cost-related insulin underuse among patients with diabetes. JAMA Intern Med. 2019;179(1):112–4. https://doi.org/10.1001/jamainternmed.2018.5008.
185. Conner F, Pfiester E, Elliott J, Slama-Chaudhry A. Unaffordable insulin: patients pay the price. Lancet Diabetes Endocrinol. 2019;7(10):748. https://doi.org/10.1016/S2213-8587(19)30260-8.
186. Hernandez I, San-Juan-Rodriguez A, Good CB, Gellad WF. Changes in list prices, net prices, and discounts for branded drugs in the US, 2007-2018. JAMA. 2020;323(9):854–62. https://doi.org/10.1001/jama.2020.1012.
187. NovoNordisk. 2023. Novopen® 6 and Novopen Echo® Plus. Accessed September 12, 2023. https://www.novonordisk.com/our-products/smart-pens/novopen-6.html.
188. Lilly.com | Eli Lilly and Company. www.lilly.com. 2023. Accessed September 1, 2023. https://www.lilly.com/resources/insulin-affordability.
189. Sanofi. Sanofi capping its insulin to a $35 out-of-pocket costs in the U.S. www.sanofi.com. 2023. Published June 1, 2023. Accessed September 15, 2023. https://www.sanofi.com/en/investors/environment-social-governance/latest-news/sanofi-capping-its-insulin-to-a-35-out-of-pocket-costs-in-the-us.

Chapter 3
Understanding Continuous Glucose Monitoring

Renee Murray-Bachmann, Ramya Pendyaia, Teresa Cichosz, Erwin Yeung, and Sarah Fishman

Introduction

Continuous glucose monitors (CGMs) have emerged as indispensable tools in diabetes management, proving beneficial across outpatient and inpatient settings alike. Effective glycemic control is pivotal in mitigating the morbidity and mortality associated with extreme glucose fluctuations, encompassing both hypoglycemia and hyperglycemia, as well as the diverse microvascular and macrovascular complications intrinsic diabetes mellitus (DM) [1, 2]. While conventional methods like hemoglobin A1c (HbA1c) and point-of-care testing (POCT) through capillary blood glucose measurements offer insights into glycemic status, their scope remains limited. HbA1c, serving as a 3-month average of blood glucose levels, fails to capture the nuances of glycemic variability. Moreover, its accuracy can be compromised in individuals with conditions like anemia, renal diseases, hemoglobinopathies, and other comorbidities due to fluctuations in hemoglobin molecule concentrations and turnover. Similarly, capillary blood glucose measurements offer only a snapshot of

R. Murray-Bachmann (✉)
Department of Nursing, Lenox Hill Hospital, Northwell Health, New York, NY, USA
e-mail: rmurraybac@northwell.edu

R. Pendyaia
Forest Hills Hospital, Northwell Health, Forest Hills, NY, USA
e-mail: rpendyala@northwell.edu

T. Cichosz
Glen Cove Hospital, Northwell Health, Glen Cove, NY, USA
e-mail: tcichosz@northwell.edu

E. Yeung · S. Fishman
Lenox Hill Hospital, Northwell Health, New York, NY, USA
e-mail: Eyeung@northwell.edu; Sfishman13@northwell.edu

S. Fishman (ed.), *Advances in Diabetes Technology*, Contemporary Endocrinology, https://doi.org/10.1007/978-3-031-75352-7_3

glucose levels at a specific moment in time and may not accurately represent glycemic trends, especially during rapid fluctuations. This limitation can be particularly burdensome for patients on insulin regimens, who are advised to check their glucose levels frequently. The discomfort associated with frequent fingerstick measurements can lead to non-compliance with monitoring regimens.

Continuous glucose monitoring systems (CGMs) offer a less invasive alternative to traditional glucose meters, potentially improving adherence to monitoring protocols and facilitating more precise and personalized diabetes management strategies. These devices continuously monitor blood glucose levels, providing real-time data on glucose dynamics throughout the day and night, thereby empowering both patients and healthcare providers in optimizing glycemic control and improving patient outcomes. Several studies have shown that use of CGMs positively impacts A1c levels, in patients with uncontrolled diabetes mellitus [3]. CGMs consist of wearable or implantable devices, with wearable options typically comprising an external transmitter and a small catheter inserted subcutaneously. Implantable devices, on the other hand, feature a long-lived sensor placed subcutaneously, with a removable and rechargeable external transmitter.

Wearable CGM devices consist of an external transmitter and a small catheter inserted into the subcutaneous space. These devices can be comfortably placed on various areas of the body such as the arm, upper thigh, flank, or abdomen. Patients typically self-apply and remove these devices, with replacements required every 7–14 days. On the other hand, implantable CGM devices feature a long-lived sensor placed subcutaneously, accompanied by a removable and rechargeable external transmitter. The implantable portion of these devices can remain in place for up to 6 months although insertion and removal of the sensor necessitate a small incision into the arm. Glucose measurements from both types of devices are transmitted via Bluetooth or near-field communication to a receiver device or smartphone for monitoring and analysis. These may require calibration and may require the use of POCT for confirmation of extreme glucose values [4].

Types of CGM Devices

1. **Intermittently Scanned (is-CGM):** These patient-owned devices continuously measure glucose levels but require intermittent scanning with a reader or smartphone for visualization and storage of glucose values [4, 5].
2. **Real-Time CGMs (rt-CGM):** These devices continuously measure and display glucose levels without requiring additional intervention from the patient once inserted and primed. Once synchronized with a phone application or reader, users can easily view their glucose levels at any time as long as the reader or phone is within 30 feet of the user.

3. **Professional CGM:** These clinic-owned devices are used by healthcare providers and may be provided to patients for temporary monitoring. They are typically worn for 5–14 days and can provide valuable glucose data for assessment. Data obtained from these devices may or may not be available in real time to the patient [4–7]

   Examples include:

   - **FreeStyle Libre Pro:** This device offers an ambulatory glucose profile reflecting 14 days of data. The provider maintains the reader in their office and can scan multiple patients. Readings are not available to the user in real time.
   - **Medtronic iPro2:** This device records glucose results every 5 min using a small, lightweight, and watertight continuous glucose monitor. The sensor is worn for up to 6 days and then returned to the provider for data downloading and assessment, with readings not available to the user in real time.

There are a number of personal continuous glucose monitors, presently available for use. The examples are included in Table 3.1.

   - **Dexcom G6 Pro:** Similar to the Medtronic device, the Dexcom G6 Pro is worn continuously by patients during their daily activities. After 7 days, the patient returns the sensor to the provider for data downloading and analysis.

Table 3.1 Currently available types of glucose monitors

Name	Wear time	Unit type
FreeStyle Libre professional and personal	14 days	All in one
FreeStyle Libre 2	14 days	All in one
FreeStyle Libre 2 plus	15 days	All in one
FreeStyle Libre 3	14 days	All in one
Dexcom Professional and G5	7 days	2-part unit transmitter reusable
Dexcom G6	10 days	2-part unit transmitter reusable
Dexcom G7	10 days	All in one
Dexcom Stelo (over the counter)	10 days	All in one
Medtronic I-pro2-Professional CGM	7 days	Returned to provider
Medtronic Guardian 3	7 days	2-part unit transmitter reusable
Medtronic Guardian 4	7 days	2-part unit transmitter reusable
Medtronic Enlite	7 days	2-part unit transmitter reusable
Medtronic Simplera	7 days	All in one
Eversense	6 months	Implantable sensor-transmitter reusable

However, readings can be made available to the user in real time, providing immediate insights into their glycemic status.

FreeStyle Libre

Abbott's FreeStyle Libre line offers a range of sensors designed to revolutionize glucose monitoring for individuals with diabetes. Among the most popular variants are the Libre 2, Libre 2 Pro, and Libre 3 sensors. The Libre 2 sensors feature a discreet small white disc, roughly the size of three stacked quarters, housing a tiny catheter inserted into the subcutaneous space on the back of the upper arm. This catheter is connected to an external transmitter affixed to the skin surface. Utilizing near-field communication technology, users can scan the external sensor using a smartphone or dedicated reader device to access glucose values. Glucose levels are calculated every 5 min, but they are only displayed when the sensor is scanned. The sensors have the capacity to store and transmit up to 8 h of data when scanned, providing users with insights into their glucose trends over time. One of the key features of the Libre 2 sensors is their built-in alarms, which can alert users to both low and high glucose values, prompting timely action. These sensors require replacement every 14 days, ensuring continuous monitoring and data collection.

It is important to note that the Libre 2 sensors do not inherently communicate or integrate data with insulin pumps. However, a modified version, the Libre 2 Pro, has recently been approved and is now available for integration with Tandem insulin pump systems. Unlike the standard Libre 2 sensors, the Libre 2 Pro does not require scanning and can provide real-time visualization of glucose values, offering enhanced convenience and usability.

The latest addition to the FreeStyle Libre lineup is the Libre 3 device, which also offers real-time visualization of glucose values. Notably, the Libre 3 is even smaller than its predecessor, approximately the size of two stacked pennies, further enhancing comfort and discretion for users [8].

Dexcom [9]

Currently, Dexcom offers two continuous glucose monitoring (CGM) systems, each designed to provide individuals with diabetes real-time insights into their glucose levels. The Dexcom G6 system is comprised of three main components: sensor, transmitter, reader or smartphone. The sensor is applied to the arm, abdomen, or leg and needs to be replaced every 10 days. It continuously measures glucose levels in the interstitial fluid. The transmitter is inserted into the sensor to transmit glucose readings wirelessly to either an external reader or a smartphone. This transmitter typically lasts up to 90 days and can be removed and reinserted when sensors are replaced. Dexcom G6 readers are available for users who prefer not to use smartphones. However, the system can also be paired with smartphones for convenient and discreet glucose monitoring. The Dexcom G6 system offers integration with Omnipod and Tandem insulin pump devices, enabling closed-loop insulin delivery systems for more precise glycemic control.

In February 2023, Dexcom released an updated version of their CGM system, the Dexcom G7. This version features a significant improvement as the sensor and transmitter are integrated into one device. Users insert and replace this device every 10 days, simplifying the system's setup and maintenance. Similar to the G6, the G7 can be paired with either an external reader or a smartphone for glucose monitoring. The Dexcom G7 is currently undergoing limited market release to integrate with Omnipod automated insulin delivery systems, expanding its compatibility and usability. This system provides real-time visualization of glucose values, accompanied by arrows indicating the direction and rate of glucose trends. Integrated alarms alert users to impending low glucose levels and critical low (<55 mg/dL) glucose events predicted within the next 20 min, allowing for prompt intervention and management.

Medtronic [10]

The Medtronic Guardian sensors offer continuous monitoring of glucose levels in the interstitial fluid, providing readings every 5 min. The sensors can be comfortably worn on either the abdomen or arm. Each sensor is paired with a transmitter, which is directly attached to the sensor. The transmitter wirelessly sends glucose information to a dedicated application on the patient's smartphone. Following a 2-h synchronization/warm-up period, real-time glucose values are displayed on the application. These values are accompanied by arrows indicating the direction and rate of glucose trends. One notable feature of the Guardian system is its predictive capabilities. The application utilizes algorithms to predict glucose trends over the next hour, allowing users to anticipate fluctuations in their glucose levels. Additionally, alarms can be set to alert users to predicted hypoglycemic or hyperglycemic events within the next 10–60 min, enabling proactive management and intervention.

While the Guardian sensors can be used as standalone devices, they are commonly integrated with insulin pump systems. This integration streamlines diabetes management by providing users with comprehensive data on their glucose levels and insulin delivery, ultimately facilitating optimized glycemic control and improved quality of life.

Eversense [11]

The Eversense CGM system stands out from other continuous glucose monitors (CGMs). Unlike traditional CGM systems, Eversense comprises an implantable sensor with an impressive lifetime of up to 6 months. This sensor is surgically implanted into the subcutaneous space of the arm through a small incision. The system's external transmitter is placed directly on the skin above the implanted sensor. This transmitter facilitates real-time visualization of glucose values without the need for an external reader device. What sets Eversense apart is that the transmitter can be removed and replaced at the user's discretion, without necessitating re-implantation of the sensor. This feature may be attractive to users who are faced with situations where they would like to avoid visual evidence of CGM use (e.g., at parties or events, or for individuals undergoing religious bathing immersions). The Eversense system also offers a novel approach to alerts for low and high glucose events. Instead of relying on audible alarms or external readers, the transmitter utilizes unique vibration patterns to alert the user to impending glycemic fluctuations. This discreet alert system provides users with valuable information while maintaining privacy and discretion. Overall, the Eversense CGM system offers a unique combination of long-term sensor implantation, flexible transmitter usage, and discreet alert mechanisms, making it an attractive option for individuals seeking both effective glucose monitoring and minimal external visibility of their CGM use.

Randomized Controlled Trials Evaluating Continuous Glucose Monitoring

Several randomized controlled trials (RCTs) have investigated the efficacy of real-time continuous glucose monitoring (rtCGM) devices in individuals with both type 1 and type 2 diabetes, with predominantly positive outcomes regarding glycemic control and hypoglycemia prevention.

Type 1 Diabetes

RCTs involving adults and youth with type 1 diabetes using continuous subcutaneous insulin infusion (CSII) or multiple daily injections (MDI) have consistently shown reductions in A1C levels and hypoglycemic episodes with regular rtCGM device usage. Studies have demonstrated significant benefits across various age groups, including seniors. However, data in children have been less consistent, with some studies showing positive outcomes while others have not [12, 13].

Type 2 Diabetes

RCTs in individuals with type 2 diabetes, particularly those on MDI or mixed therapies, have also reported reductions in A1C levels following rtCGM use. However, the reduction in hypoglycemia rates has not been as consistently observed compared to type 1 diabetes populations. Notably, these improvements in glycemic control have occurred without significant changes in insulin doses or other diabetes medications.

Intermittently Scanned Continuous Glucose Monitoring (isCGM)

RCT data on intermittently scanned continuous glucose monitoring (isCGM) devices are more limited compared to rtCGM. Studies in adults with type 1 diabetes have shown reductions in hypoglycemia rates, while those in adults with type 2 diabetes have reported mixed outcomes regarding A1C reduction and hypoglycemia prevention. However, isCGM devices have been associated with improvements in treatment satisfaction scores in some studies.

Youth Population

RCTs involving youth with type 1 diabetes have yielded variable results, with some studies showing no significant reduction in A1C levels but indicating increased frequency of testing and improved treatment satisfaction with device usage.

Conclusion

Overall, RCTs evaluating continuous glucose monitoring devices, particularly rtCGM, have demonstrated significant benefits in improving glycemic control and reducing hypoglycemia rates, especially in individuals with type 1 diabetes. While data for type 2 diabetes and isCGM devices are more limited and mixed, there is growing evidence supporting their efficacy in certain patient populations. Further research and larger scale studies are warranted to elucidate the long-term benefits and optimal use of continuous glucose monitoring in diverse patient populations.

Accuracy of CGMs Relative to Blood Glucose Measurements

The accuracy of Continuous Glucose Monitoring (CGM) devices can be evaluated using several metrics, including the Mean Absolute Relative Difference (MARD), Clarke Error Grid Analysis, and the percentage of readings within certain predefined ranges.

Mean Absolute Relative Difference (MARD) [14, 15]

MARD is a commonly used metric that represents the average percentage difference between CGM readings and reference measurements obtained from laboratory blood tests via venipuncture. A lower MARD value indicates a more accurate CGM device [15]. For instance, a MARD of less than 10% is generally deemed acceptable for use in inpatient settings, provided there are no specific concerns about physiological conditions affecting the composition of interstitial fluid (ISF) in critically ill patients [16–18].

Clarke Error Grid Analysis

Clarke Error Grid Analysis is a graphical method designed to assess the clinical impact of CGM accuracy. This analysis involves collecting paired glucose values from the CGM device and a reference measurement method. These paired data points are then categorized into different zones based on the clinical significance of the discrepancies between CGM readings and reference values [14, 15]. The zones range from no effect, benign effect, to various levels of clinical risk. A CGM device is considered more accurate if a higher percentage of its data points fall into zones indicating no or benign clinical effects.

Percentage of Readings within Specific Ranges

Another method to evaluate CGM accuracy is by examining the percentage of CGM readings that fall within certain ranges compared to reference measurements. For example, a CGM system might be assessed based on the proportion of its readings that are within ±15 mg/dL or ±20% of the reference values. This approach provides a straightforward measure of how closely CGM readings align with actual blood glucose levels.

Overall, these metrics collectively help in determining the reliability and clinical usefulness of CGM devices. Accurate CGM devices are crucial for effective diabetes management, as they provide real-time glucose monitoring, allowing for timely adjustments in therapy and better overall glycemic control.

Table 3.2 [19] discusses the studies comparing the accuracy of CGMs (FreeStyle Libre or Dexcom G6) against FDA-approved POCT devices in the inpatient setting [19].

Table 3.2 Studies comparing the accuracy of CGM systems with a comparator [19] (Spanakis et al., 2023, used by permission of D, Klonoff MD)

Study	Year	Population	CGM type	Comparator	Outcome
Non-ICU studies					
Galindo et al.	2020	T2D, non-critically ill	FreeStyle Libre Pro	Capillary by POC	MARD 14.8%; Increased detection of asymptomatic and prolonged hypoglycemia
Migdal et al.	2020	T1D and T2D undergoing radiological procedures ($n = 49$)	Dexcom G6	Capillary by POC	MARD: 13.3% pre-imaging, 12.7% post-imaging; CEG: zones A + B 98.1% pre-imaging, 99.7% post-imaging
Tripyla et al.	2020	Prediabetes, T1D, T2D, and pancreatic diabetes undergoing abdominal surgery ($n = 20$)	Dexcom G6	Capillary by POC	MARD: 12.7%; CEG: zones A + B 99.2%
Reutrakul et al.	2020	COVID-19 on SC insulin ($n = 9$)	Dexcom G6	Capillary by POC	MARD: 9.77%; CEG: zones A + B 100%
Nair et al.	2020	Diabetes, surgical ward ($n = 10$)	Dexcom G6 blinded	Capillary by POC	MARD: 9.4%; CEG: zones A + B 89%
Davis et al.	2021	Non-critically ill, 96% T2D ($n = 298$)	Dexcom G6	Capillary by POC	MARD 12.8%; CEG: zones A + B 98.7%
Murray-Bachmann et al.	2021	Diabetes, non-critically ill ($n = 52$)	FreeStyle Libre	Capillary by POC and serum glucose	Capillary: MARD 15.6%; Serum glucose: MARD 13.2%
Longo et al.	2022	COVID-19 general floor ($n = 18$) or ICU ($n = 10$)	Dexcom G6	Capillary by POC or blood glucose analyzed in lab	MARD: 13.2% (vs. POC 13.9%; vs. lab 10.9%)
ICU studies					
Schierenbeck et al.	2017	Cardiac ICU ($n = 26$)	FreeStyle Libre	Arterial by blood gas analyzer and capillary by POC	CEG: zones A and B 99.1%

(continued)

Table 3.2 (continued)

Study	Year	Population	CGM type	Comparator	Outcome
Ancona et al.	2017	ICU (*n* = 8)	FreeStyle Libre	Arterial by blood gas analyzer and capillary by POC	MARD 14%; CEG: zones A and B 97.8%
Sadhu et al.	2020	ICU (*n* = 11)	Guardian Connect, Dexcom G6	Capillary by POC	Guardian Connect: MARD 13.1%, CEG: zones A and B 100%; Dexcom G6: MARD 11.1%; CEG: zones A and B 98%
Agarwal et al.	2021	ICU (*n* = 11)	Dexcom G6	Capillary by POC	MARD 12.58%; CEG: zones A and B 98.2%
Pérez-Guzman et al.	2021	OR Cardiac ICU (*n* = 15)	Dexcom G6 blinded	Capillary by POC	MARD 12.9%; CEG: zones A and B 98.6%
Faulds et al.	2021	COVID ICU (*n* = 18)	Dexcom G6	Capillary by POC	MARD 13.9%
Huang et al.	2022	ICU (*n* = 122)	FreeStyle Libre Pro	Venous by blood glucose lactic acid analyzer	MARD 18%; CEG: zones A and B 98.5%
Tingsarat et al.	2022	MICU (*n* = 12)	Medtronic Enlite	Capillary and plasma glucose	Capillary: MARD 6.6%; CEG zones A + B 99.7%; Plasma glucose: MARD 8.8%; CEG zones A + B 95.2%
Boeder et al.	2022	Critically ill COVID-19 (*n* = 24)	Dexcom G6	Capillary by POC	MARD 14.8%; CEG: zones A + B 99.5%
Sweeney et al.	2022	Diabetes, cardiac surgery (*n* = 11)	Dexcom G6	Capillary by POC	MARD 14.8% (12.3% for those with eGFR ≥20 mL/min/1.73 m^2); CEG: zones A and B 97%
Herzig et al.	2023	Diabetes, cardiac surgery (*n* = 16)	Dexcom G6	Arterial blood glucose by Accu-Check Inform II meter	Intrasurgery MARD 23.8%; Post-surgery MARD 15%; MARD 29.1% during hypothermic extracorporeal circulation, and 41.6% after deep hypothermic circulatory arrest

CEG clark error grid, *CGM* continuous glucose monitor, *eGFR* estimated glomerular filtration rate, *ICU* intensive care unit, *MARD* mean absolute relative difference, *MICU* medical intensive care unit, *POC* point-of-care (used with permission from D. Klonoff MD)

Discussion

MARD values for CGM systems can vary widely, ranging from 6.9% to 22.8%, depending on the specific device and the physiological conditions of the patient. These variations are particularly notable under different glycemic states:

- **Hypoglycemic Conditions**: MARD values range from 16.2% to 46.8%, indicating a higher margin of error when glucose levels are low.
- **Euglycemic Conditions**: MARD values range from 8.5% to 24%, showing moderate accuracy during normal blood glucose levels.
- **Hyperglycemic Conditions**: MARD values range from 5.1% to 15.7%, suggesting better accuracy when glucose levels are high.

For instance, a study involving the Dexcom G6 CGM system examined the device's performance during exercise. The results indicated that the MARD values did not show significant changes from pre- to post-exercise. Specifically, the MARD for aerobic exercise ranged from 8.9% to 13.9%, and for resistance exercise, it ranged from 7.7% to 14.5%. This consistency suggests that the Dexcom G6 maintains its accuracy even under physical exertion, providing reliable glucose readings for users engaged in various types of exercise.

Understanding the variability of MARD under different conditions is crucial for clinicians and patients alike. It highlights the importance of considering the specific context in which a CGM device is used. For example:

- **In Clinical Settings**: Clinicians should be aware that CGM accuracy may decrease during hypoglycemic episodes, which could impact treatment decisions. Therefore, supplementary blood glucose tests might be necessary during such times.
- **For Patients**: Knowing that their CGM device might be less accurate during hypoglycemia can prompt users to verify critical readings with a fingerstick test, particularly when symptoms of low blood sugar are present.

Additionally, the impact of physical activity on CGM performance is a key consideration for active individuals. The Dexcom G6 study demonstrates that users can rely on their CGM for accurate readings even during and after exercise, which is essential for managing exercise-induced glucose fluctuations.

The data demonstrates that the accuracy of CGM systems can vary based on the type of CGM used, the clinical setting, and the specific conditions of the patient. Generally, MARD values are lower (indicating higher accuracy) in non-ICU settings compared to ICU settings, where factors like critical illness can influence CGM performance.

Non-ICU Studies [19]

- **Galindo et al. (2020)** observed a MARD of 14.8% with the FreeStyle Libre Pro in non-critically ill patients with T2D, highlighting its utility in detecting asymptomatic and prolonged hypoglycemia.

- **et al. (2020)** reported MARD values for the Dexcom G6 before and after radiological procedures, showing high accuracy (13.3% pre-imaging, 12.7% post-imaging).
- **Tripyla et al.** [20] and **Davis et al. (2021)** demonstrated consistent accuracy with the Dexcom G6 in various patient populations undergoing surgery or in non-critically ill settings, with MARD values around 12.7% and 12.8%, respectively.
- **Reutrakul et al. (2020)** showed a notably lower MARD of 9.77% in COVID-19 patients on SC insulin, suggesting excellent performance even under the stress of infection.
- **Longo et al. (2022)** provided a comparative analysis, showing slight differences in MARD values when comparing capillary and lab glucose analyses.

ICU Studies [19]
- **Schierenbeck et al.** [10] and **Ancona et al. (2017)** focused on the FreeStyle Libre in ICU settings, with MARD around 14%, and high percentages of data in CEG zones A and B.
- **Sadhu et al. (2020)** compared Guardian Connect and Dexcom G6, both showing high accuracy with MARD values around 11–13% and CEG zones A and B close to 100%.
- **Faulds et al. (2021)** and **Huang et al. (2022)** indicated that while ICU settings pose challenges, CGMs like Dexcom G6 and FreeStyle Libre Pro maintain reasonable accuracy.
- **Herzig et al. (2023)** highlighted the significant variability in MARD during specific ICU conditions, such as hypothermic extracorporeal circulation, emphasizing the impact of extreme physiological changes on CGM accuracy.

Overall, this detailed analysis underscores the importance of considering the specific CGM device, clinical setting, and patient condition when evaluating CGM accuracy. Continuous improvements in CGM technology aim to enhance reliability, making these devices invaluable tools for diabetes management across diverse clinical scenarios.

Drawbacks to CGM Use

While Continuous Glucose Monitoring (CGM) systems offer numerous benefits for managing diabetes, there are several drawbacks that patients may encounter:

1. **Device Inconvenience and Comfort:** Patients may find CGMs inconvenient due to the need to wear the device continuously. Although many users report that these devices are generally comfortable, some individuals experience issues such as contact dermatitis caused by the adhesives used to secure the sensors. Additionally, the physical presence of the device can be uncomfortable during activities such as exercise or sleep, potentially disrupting daily routines and rest.

2. **Insurance Coverage and Affordability:** Despite their proven benefits, CGMs are not always covered by insurance plans, particularly for individuals who do not require insulin injections. This lack of coverage can be a significant barrier to access, especially for low-income individuals [18]. The out-of-pocket cost of CGM devices and the associated supplies can be prohibitive, limiting their use to those who can afford them without insurance support.
3. **Potential for Inaccurate Readings:** Certain substances can interfere with CGM readings, leading to potential inaccuracies. For example:

   - **FreeStyle Libre 2**: Ingestion of high doses of vitamin C (greater than 500 mg) and hydroxyurea can cause false readings of hyperglycemia [11]. This can mislead users into thinking their glucose levels are higher than they actually are.
   - **Eversense CGM**: The accuracy of readings can be affected by the use of mannitol and tetracycline. These substances can alter the sensor's performance, resulting in misleading glucose measurements [11].

These inaccuracies can lead to inappropriate treatment decisions, such as unnecessary insulin administration or dietary changes, potentially exacerbating the patient's condition rather than improving it.

Beyond the primary concerns mentioned, there are additional drawbacks to CGM use that patients and healthcare providers should be aware of:

1. **Calibration Requirements**: Some CGM systems require regular calibration with fingerstick blood glucose tests to ensure accuracy. This additional step can be burdensome for users, detracting from the convenience that CGMs are supposed to offer.
2. **Learning Curve and User Education**: Proper use of CGM technology involves a learning curve. Users need to be educated on how to interpret the data, respond to alerts, and adjust their treatment plans accordingly. Without adequate training, the benefits of CGMs may not be fully realized, and there is a risk of misuse or over-reliance on the device.
3. **Technical Issues and Reliability**: CGM devices can occasionally malfunction or experience technical issues, such as sensor errors or connectivity problems with associated apps and devices. These technical glitches can disrupt monitoring and lead to periods without glucose data, which can be particularly problematic for users who rely heavily on CGMs for real-time glucose management.
4. **Emotional and Psychological Impact**: The constant awareness of glucose levels and the frequent alerts from CGM devices can contribute to anxiety and stress for some users. The pressure to maintain optimal glucose levels and the fear of hypoglycemia or hyperglycemia can be overwhelming, potentially impacting mental health.
5. **Skin Reactions and Long-term Use**: Prolonged use of CGM sensors can lead to skin reactions beyond contact dermatitis, such as skin irritation, rashes, or infections at the insertion site. Managing these skin issues can be challenging and may necessitate discontinuing CGM use, which can disrupt diabetes management.

In conclusion, while CGM systems provide invaluable benefits for diabetes management, including better glucose control and reduced hospital admissions, they are not without drawbacks. Patients may face issues with device convenience, comfort, and affordability, as well as potential inaccuracies due to interfering substances. Additionally, there are challenges related to calibration, user education, technical reliability, emotional impact, and skin reactions. Addressing these concerns through improved device design, better insurance coverage, comprehensive user training, and ongoing support can help maximize the benefits of CGMs and enhance the quality of life for diabetes patients.

Assessment of Glycemic Control

The Diabetes Technology Society emphasizes the importance of monitoring Time Below Range (TBR), Time in Range (TIR), and Time Above Range (TAR) in both percentage and total minutes for individuals using CGMs [19]. These metrics are invaluable for assessing glycemic control. According to Bellido et al., these target glucose ranges should be individualized to optimize diabetes management.

Time in Range (TIR) and Glycemic Control

Multiple studies comparing glycemic control between individuals using POCT devices and CGMs have demonstrated that TIR is significantly greater in those using CGMs. This corroborates existing literature showing that CGMs are effective in decreasing hypoglycemic events. The continuous data provided by CGMs allows for a more comprehensive understanding of glucose trends and facilitates timely interventions, reducing the risk of acute complications.

CGMs vs. POCT in Inpatient Settings

The FDA-approved platform for inpatient glucose testing is currently POCT devices. However, CGMs offer several advantages, including the ability to monitor glucose trends continuously, with readings every 5 min over periods ranging from 10 to 14 days, depending on the device. For example, the Eversense implantable sensor lasts for up to 6 months [21]. This continuous monitoring can significantly decrease the incidence of acute complications such as hypo- and hyperglycemia due to timely interventions that would not be possible with a single real-time glucose result.

Benefits for Specific Populations

CGMs have proven particularly beneficial for certain populations, including those with Type 1 Diabetes Mellitus, the elderly, and individuals with conditions such as insulinoma, Hirata disease, and cystic fibrosis. The technology's ability to provide glucose trending alarms and alerts for acute complications makes it especially efficacious for these groups [22–24].

Limitations of POCT in Critical Care

In hospitalized patients, glucose POCT is typically ordered pre-meal, at bedtime, and at additional times when correctional insulin doses are needed. Critical care patients on continuous insulin infusions, such as those being treated for diabetic ketoacidosis, often require hourly POCT. Despite frequent monitoring, the intervals between tests can allow unmonitored trends towards hypo- or hyperglycemia. Inpatient hypoglycemia is defined as blood glucose values below 70 mg/dL (below 60 mg/dL in prenatal patients), with critical results below 54 mg/dL now being a CMS reportable measure. The use of CGMs in inpatient settings can help avoid these extreme glycemic excursions by providing continuous data.

Regulatory Changes and Integration Challenges

With the onset of the COVID-19 pandemic, the FDA granted a waiver in April 2020 allowing the use of CGMs in inpatient settings [19, 25]. This waiver facilitated remote monitoring of blood glucose levels by healthcare staff, thereby reducing exposure to the virus. As of March 1, 2022, the FDA has provided Breakthrough Device Designation for Dexcom CGM technology for use in hospital settings and does not intend to object to the continued distribution of Dexcom CGMs to hospitals.

However, this does not eliminate the need for POCT devices, which remain the FDA-approved platform and are easily synchronized with Electronic Medical Records (EMR). A significant challenge to the widespread adoption of CGMs in inpatient settings is the integration and documentation within existing EHR systems [19, 25]. Informatics updates are necessary to incorporate CGM data effectively into the EMR. Currently, guidelines for the analysis and documentation of CGM data in inpatient settings are not standardized. The Diabetes Technology Society has proposed standards for integrating CGM data into the EMR, which will be crucial for the widespread adoption of this technology.

CGMs represent a significant advancement in the management of diabetes, offering continuous, real-time glucose monitoring that can greatly improve glycemic control. The metrics of TBR, TIR, and TAR are essential for assessing the effectiveness of CGMs. While CGMs have proven beneficial for outpatient use, their integration into inpatient settings poses challenges, particularly regarding EHR compatibility and documentation standards. Addressing these challenges will be crucial for leveraging the full potential of CGM technology in both outpatient and inpatient diabetes management.

Core Data Set for EHR Documentation

The core data set for Electronic Health Record (EHR) documentation, as outlined by the Diabetes Technology Society, includes comprehensive metrics essential for managing diabetes with Continuous Glucose Monitoring (CGM) systems. This table provides a comparison between the iCoDE core data set and hospital-specific core data set, highlighting the necessary parameters for effective diabetes management and monitoring (Table 3.3).

Table 3.3 Core data set for EHR documentation [19] Spanakis et al., 2023, used by permission of D. Klonoff MD

iCoDE Core data set	Hospital-specific core data set
• Mean glucose	• Mean glucose
• Glucose management indicator (GMI)	—
• Glycemic variability (% CV)	• Glycemic variability (%CV)
• Time above range, very high (% time >250 mg/dL)	• Time above range, very high (% time >250 mg/dL)
• Time above range, high (% time 180–250 mg/dL)	• Time above range, high (% time 180–250 mg/dL)
• Time in range (TIR), (% time 70–180 mg/dL)	• Time in range (TIR), (% time 70–180 mg/dL)
• Time below range, low (% time 54–69 mg/dL)	• Time below range, low (% time 54–69 mg/dL)
• Time below range, very low (% time <54 mg/dL)	• Time below range, very low (% time <54 mg/dL)
• Ambulatory Glucose Profile (AGP) Report	• Hospital Glucose Profile Report
• Individual glucose values	—
• Number of days CGM worn	• Number of days CGM worn
• Percentage of time CGM is active	• Percentage of time CGM is active
• CGM reporting period start/end dates	• CGM reporting period start/end dates
• CGM manufacturer name and model	• CGM manufacturer name and model
—	• Glycemia risk index (GRI)

CGM continuous glucose monitor, *CV* coefficient of variability, *GMI* glucose management indicator, *GRI* glycemia risk index, *TAR* time above range, *TBR* time below range, *TIR* time in range (table used with permission from D. Klonoff MD)

Clinical Contraindications for the Use of CGMS

Continuous Glucose Monitoring Systems (CGMS) have proven beneficial for many patients managing diabetes. However, there are specific clinical settings and conditions where their use is contraindicated or limited due to concerns regarding accuracy and safety. This includes certain critical care environments and during specific medical procedures.

CGM systems are not currently approved for use in intensive care units (ICUs) due to concerns about their accuracy in critically ill patients. Specific conditions that affect CGM accuracy in these settings include hypotension, hypoxemia, acidosis, anasarca, and vasoconstriction [19, 25, 26]. These conditions can significantly alter interstitial fluid (ISF) composition, affecting CGM readings .

Medical Imaging and Procedures

Initially, the impact of various medical imaging modalities on CGM functionality was a concern, leading to recommendations that CGMs be removed prior to these procedures. Recent studies have updated these guidelines based on new evidence:

1. **Ultrasound, X-ray, and CT Scans**:
   - CGMs can remain in place during these procedures.
   - These tests do not impact sensor accuracy.
   - Lead shields are not required, as they can necessitate higher radiation doses.
   - Patients should verify CGM readings against a glucose meter for at least 2 h post-procedure.
2. **MRI Scans**:
   - CGMs like the Eversense [8, 11] can remain functional post-MRI under specific conditions: static magnetic fields of 1.5 T or 3 T, with a maximum spatial field gradient of 4000 g/cm (40 T/m).
   - Despite this, hospitals generally maintain the policy of removing CGMs before MRI scans to avoid complications due to possible non-adherence to these specific magnetic field conditions.

Procedures Requiring CGM Removal

As of 2024, CGMs should be removed prior to the following procedures due to potential risks and unknown effects [8–11].

1. **Lithotripsy**:
   - This ultrasound shock wave treatment can potentially damage inserted sensors, such as Eversense, due to unknown effects on the device [14].
2. **Diathermy**:
   - The generation of heat using electrical pulses can transfer energy through the sensor, causing tissue damage at the insertion site [14].
3. **Electrocautery**:
   - This involves using a heated electrode to stop blood flow or destroy tissue and may damage the CGM device. Abbott Diabetes Care notes that electrocautery has not been tested with FreeStyle Libre Systems, but potential risks include interference with the sensor's electrical components [14].
4. **Electrosurgery**:
   - This group of procedures uses high-frequency alternating electrical current for tissue destruction (including electrocoagulation, electrofulguration, electrodesiccation, and electrosection). Electrosurgery can produce electromagnetic interference, potentially disrupting CGM functionality [14].

While CGMs are highly beneficial for many patients, there are significant contraindications in certain clinical settings and during specific procedures. These include critical care environments where physiological conditions can affect CGM accuracy, as well as during certain medical imaging and therapeutic procedures due to potential risks to device functionality and patient safety. Adhering to guidelines and removing CGMs when necessary helps ensure both the accuracy of glucose monitoring and patient safety.

Evidence Supporting the Outpatient Use of CGMs

Aggarwal et al. published a comprehensive review of 12 studies evaluating the impact of CGMs on healthcare spending and clinical outcomes in patients with Type 1 and Type 2 diabetes mellitus. Out of these studies, seven were retrospective. The review revealed significant cost savings and clinical benefits associated with the use of CGMs compared to Point-of-Care Testing (POCT).

1. **Cost Savings:** The review found that the total healthcare cost, including medications, equipment, and medical interventions, was markedly lower for CGM users compared to those relying on POCT ($16,194 vs $20,452). This cost reduction is attributed to the improved ability of CGM users to monitor and manage their

glucose levels more effectively. By providing continuous and real-time glucose data, CGMs enable users to identify trends in hypoglycemia and hyperglycemia, allowing for timely interventions that prevent acute complications and reduce the need for hospital admissions.

2. **Reduction in Hospital Admissions:** One of the significant findings of the review was the reduction in hospital admissions related to diabetes complications. CGM usage was associated with fewer admissions for diabetic ketoacidosis (DKA), non-DKA hyperglycemia, and hypoglycemia. This reduction is likely due to the enhanced capability of CGMs to detect and alert users to abnormal glucose levels, enabling them to take corrective actions before acute complications develop.
3. **Improved Daily Functioning:** The review also highlighted the positive impact of CGM usage on daily functioning. Users of CGMs experienced significant reductions in employment and school absenteeism. By maintaining better glucose control and preventing severe glucose fluctuations, CGM users are less likely to experience debilitating episodes that require time off from work or school [27].

The evidence supporting the outpatient use of CGMs extends beyond just cost savings and reduced hospital admissions. CGMs provide several additional benefits that contribute to the overall health and well-being of diabetes patients:

1. **Improved Glycemic Control**: CGMs offer real-time glucose monitoring, which helps patients and healthcare providers make more informed decisions regarding insulin dosing and lifestyle adjustments. This can lead to better long-term glycemic control and reduce the risk of diabetes-related complications.
2. **Enhanced Quality of Life**: The continuous feedback from CGMs can alleviate the anxiety associated with unpredictable glucose levels, improving the quality of life for diabetes patients. Knowing their glucose levels at all times can empower patients to engage more confidently in daily activities, including exercise and social events.
3. **Personalized Diabetes Management**: CGMs allow for personalized diabetes management by providing detailed glucose data that can be used to tailor treatment plans. This individualized approach can help optimize insulin therapy and dietary choices, further enhancing glycemic control.
4. **Patient Education and Engagement**: The use of CGMs can serve as an educational tool for patients, helping them understand the impact of different foods, activities, and medications on their glucose levels. Increased awareness and engagement in their own care can lead to more proactive and effective diabetes management.
5. **Integration with Other Technologies**: Many CGMs can be integrated with insulin pumps and smartphone applications, creating a seamless diabetes management system. This integration can provide comprehensive data analytics and trend reports, further aiding in effective diabetes management.

Overall, the review by Aggarwal et al. underscores the numerous advantages of CGMs in outpatient settings, from economic benefits to improved health outcomes and quality of life for diabetes patients. As CGM technology continues to advance, it is expected to play an increasingly vital role in the management of diabetes, making it a valuable tool for both patients and healthcare providers.

Using CGM in the Inpatient Setting

Clinical Professional Staff Instructions for CGM Use in Hospitalized Patients

General Instructions

1. **Confirming Hypoglycemia:**
   - When CGM indicates hypoglycemia, confirm the reading with a hospital-approved Point-of-Care Testing (POCT) device before proceeding with treatment according to the hospital's hypoglycemia protocol [19, 26].
   - If the patient's symptoms do not match the CGM readings, use the POCT device to ensure accuracy.
2. **Addressing CGM Malfunctions:**
   - If the CGM sensor fails to provide readings or trend arrows, obtain a glucose reading using the POCT device.
3. **Situations Requiring POCT Use in Addition to CGM** [28]**:**
   - After physiotherapy
   - Post-severe hypotension
   - Post-surgery
   - After cardiac arrest

CGMs measure glucose levels in interstitial fluid, while POCT devices use capillary blood, which provides more accurate glucose assessments. This is of the utmost importance as CGMs use interstitial fluid whereas the more accurate POCT uses capillary blood for glucose assessment. Furthermore, the CGM sensor results may be rendered unreliable due to temperature, hydration, rapid changes in blood glucose, and tissue perfusion. CGM must not be placed in areas of cellulitis or edema or on the side of a surgical site [28].

Analysis of CGM in the Inpatient Setting

Glycemic Control Metrics

1. **Time Below Range (TBR):**
    - Reported as percentages and in minutes for Level 1 (<70 mg/dL) and Level 2 (<54 mg/dL).
    - Calculate the percentage and minutes of CGM values below these thresholds over 1 day or the entire inpatient stay.
2. **Hypoglycemic Events:**
    - Defined as CGM values below Level 1 or Level 2 thresholds for at least 15 min.
    - Each hypoglycemic occurrence is considered a separate event.
    - Nocturnal hypoglycemic events are those occurring between 11:00 pm and 7:00 am.
3. **Recurrent Hypoglycemic Days:**
    - Percentage of days with at least one hypoglycemic event lasting at least 15 min, occurring on separate days during the hospital stay.
4. **Mild Recommendations for Recurrent Hypoglycemic Events:**
    - Another hypoglycemic event following a previous one, separated by at least 15 min without a hypoglycemic value.
5. **Prolonged Hypoglycemic Events:**
    - Number of events with hypoglycemic values lasting at least 2 h per day or per hospital admission.
6. **Time at High Risk for Hypoglycemia (THRH):**
    - Proportion of time (percentage) or number of minutes in hypoglycemia.

Hyperglycemia Metrics

1. **Definition:**
    - Sensor glucose value >180 mg/dL for at least 15 min for patients with pre-existing diabetes.
    - For those with normal glucose levels pre-admission, hyperglycemia is defined as ≥140 mg/dL.
    - Level 2 hyperglycemia is defined as >250 mg/dL lasting at least 2 h.
2. **Analysis:**
    - Monitor and report the percentage of time and the number of minutes spent in hyperglycemia.
    - Count the number of events with hyperglycemic values.

Summary

By adhering to these guidelines, clinical staff can ensure the accurate and effective use of CGMs in hospitalized patients. This involves confirming CGM readings with POCT devices when necessary, recognizing situations that necessitate additional monitoring, and understanding the impact of various conditions and procedures on CGM accuracy. Monitoring glycemic control metrics, such as TBR, hypoglycemic events, and hyperglycemia, provides valuable insights into patient outcomes and can inform adjustments in care plans to better manage diabetes in the inpatient setting.

Use of CGM Devices During Surgical Procedures

According to the ADA professional practice committee, 20% of general surgical patients have diabetes mellitus and 23–60% have undiagnosed diabetes or prediabetes [29]. Perioperative glucose control is of the utmost importance to assure adequate wound healing. Hypoglycemia engenders increased morbidity and mortality in the surgical patient living with diabetes mellitus and is a known acute complication. It is recommended that blood glucose be maintained 100–200 mg/dL (as stricter goals increase risk for hypoglycemia) but the use of point-of-care devices can allow for missed acute complications [16] The stress associated with undergoing surgical procedures leads to an increase in catecholamines, growth hormone, endogenous corticosteroids, and glucagon, while decreasing insulin secretion and increasing insulin resistance [11, 16], thus increasing hyperglycemia and the associated infection, length of stay [30] and mortality [27]. This hyperglycemia negatively impacts wound healing due to leukocyte dysregulation [31]· General anesthesia (halothane, enflurane, isoflurane) releases counterregulatory hormones which also raises glucose levels [27, 31, 32]

The use of the CGM in the perioperative areas (pre-surgical testing, ambulatory surgery, operating theater as opposed to a POCT device which are not only glucose meters, but devices such as an ISTAT, GEM5000, or awaiting the results of serum glucose) has been shown to identify hypo- and hyperglycemic trends (which can be displayed on a receiver) thus allowing for rapid intervention. Though the present standards are that CGM should not be used alone for glucose monitoring during surgery [27]; according to Price et al, hypoglycemia occurrences engender concern in anesthesia providers [33] especially when there is a delay in recognition. Furthermore, hyperglycemia may delay general anesthesia recovery. Hyperglycemia can lead to metabolic disturbances including DKA requiring intraoperative resuscitation, in addition to increasing the risk of surgical site infection, stroke, and myocardial infarction [30, 31, 34–39]

Studies Supporting CGM Use in Surgery:

- **Prospective Cohort Study:** Carlsson et al. found that CGMs identified higher proportions of hypo- and hyperglycemia during major surgery compared to POCT. .
- **Dexcom G6 Study:** A study comparing the Dexcom G6 CGM with POCT during elective abdominal surgery reported a mean absolute relative difference (MARD) of 12.7 ± 8.7%. The study found 99.2% of CGM measurements within Clarke error grid zones A and B, with CGM readings overestimating reference glucose by 1.1 ± 14.4 mg/dL.

Current Recommendations: Integrating CGM devices in the perioperative management of diabetic patients offers significant advantages by providing continuous glucose monitoring, allowing timely interventions, and improving surgical outcomes. While current standards recommend against using CGMs alone during surgery, integrating CGM with traditional POCT can enhance glucose management by providing continuous monitoring alongside intermittent POCT confirmation and can offer a comprehensive approach to managing perioperative glucose levels.

Use of CGM Devices in Pregnancy

There is growing evidence supporting the use of Continuous Glucose Monitors (CGMs) in pregnancy, particularly for women with pre-existing diabetes (Type 1 or Type 2) and those with gestational diabetes mellitus (GDM) [40, 41].

Benefits of CGM in Pregnancy:

- **Tight Glycemic Control:** Maintaining tight glycemic control during pregnancy is crucial for both maternal and fetal health [41]. CGMs provide real-time glucose monitoring, allowing for prompt adjustments to insulin therapy, diet, and lifestyle based on continuous data.
- **Minimizing Glycemic Episodes:** CGMs help in minimizing episodes of hypoglycemia and hyperglycemia, promoting a stable blood glucose environment for the developing fetus [41].
- **Improved Pregnancy Outcomes:** Studies have shown that the use of CGMs during pregnancy is associated with improved outcomes, including reduced risk of macrosomia (excessive fetal growth) and other complications. Better glucose control with CGMs has been linked to decreased risks of preterm birth, preeclampsia, and other maternal and neonatal complications [40, 41].
- **Labor and Delivery Monitoring:** Primary data from recent clinical trials indicate that CGM use during labor can identify early trends that may suggest and resolve neonatal hypoglycemia post-delivery. However, Pinson et al. suggest that more studies are indicated for CGM use during actual labor and delivery [40].

- **Insulin Drip Protocols:** In cases where insulin drip protocols are warranted (necessitating hourly glucose monitoring), CGMs may prove more efficacious than POCT, offering continuous monitoring and timely adjustments.

Case Report: CGM Use in a Critically Ill Inpatient

Patient Profile: A 40 y/o Caucasian female with history of T1DM, and end-stage renal disease on peritoneal dialysis, presented from a rehabilitation facility for evaluation of peripheral arterial disease requiring following recent knee amputation of the left lower extremity and right great toe amputation. On presentation, she was found to have sepsis. Initial bloodwork revealed a hemoglobin A1c of 8.6% which was felt to be an inaccurate reflection of patients average glycemic control due to the patients' comorbidities. The patient was started on multiple daily insulin injections, necessitating frequent blood glucose monitoring.

Given the patient's history of type 1 diabetes, she was started on a regimen of multiple daily insulin injections. As such, she required frequent blood glucose monitoring. POCT using the FDA-approved Accu-Chek II platform is the standard; however, capillary blood from alternate sites other than the finger [42] is not appropriate for testing on the Accu-Chek Inform II Meter. This patient however had gangrene of all fingers, preventing the collection of capillary glucose. The decision was therefore made to allow the use of glucose readings from the patients Dexcom G7 device to inform clinical decision-making. The patient placed a new CGM on her right arm the day before admission, which remained in place for 10 days. On day 1 of admission, 4/12/23 patient returned to the OR for further wound debridement .

Blood Glucose Results:

- **Day 1 (4/12/23):**

  10:48 – 126 mg/dL
  14:16 – 145 mg/dL
  16:59 – 198 mg/dL
  21:51 – 384 mg/dL

- **Subsequent Results:**

  05:07 – 298 mg/dL
  06:40 – 143 mg/dL
  06:56 – 86 mg/dL
  08:53 – 135 mg/dL
  14:16 – 145 mg/dL
  16:59 – 198 mg/dL

Critical Incident:

- **Code Blue:** The patient's condition deteriorated post-second procedure, resulting in a code blue being called on 4/13/2023 at 1:06 am. She was moved to the SICU, where she remained until 4/17.

Sensor Readings During Critical Period:

2:17 – 296 mg/dL
2:55 – 360 mg/dL
4:04 – 277 mg/dL
5:22 – 234 mg/dL
6:44 - 195 mg/dL
8:38 – 119 mg/dL

Follow-up Surgery: planned for 4/21/23: Elective amputation of bilateral necrotic digits of the upper extremity and right lower extremity TMA debridement.

Hypoglycemia Incident: 43 mg/dL at 10:33 on 4/13/2023, which would not have been identified without the CGM.

This case study illustrates the practical application of CGMs in the inpatient setting, especially when FDA-approved POCT platforms are not feasible. Continuous glucose monitoring provided critical insights into the patient's glycemic status, enabling timely and informed clinical decision-making.

Conclusions on CGM Usage in the Inpatient Setting

Advantages of CGM in Hospitalized Patients:

- **Early Identification of Glycemic Trends:** Continuous glucose monitors (CGMs) enable the early detection of hypoglycemic and hyperglycemic trends, allowing for timely interventions that can significantly decrease morbidity and mortality.
- **Reduction of Acute Complications:** Timely recognition and management of glycemic fluctuations can prevent acute complications, thus improving patient outcomes in critical care situations.

Limitations and Contraindications:

- **Medical Conditions:** CGMs are not recommended in certain medical conditions such as edema, cellulitis, or post-cardiac arrest scenarios, due to potential inaccuracies and complications.
- **Diagnostic Procedures:** CGMs must be removed prior to specific medical procedures, including electrosurgery and MRI, due to potential interference and safety concerns.

Future Directions and Studies Needed:

- **Technological Integration:** Further technological analysis is required to ensure CGMs can synchronize effectively with electronic medical records, enhancing data accessibility and clinical decision-making.
- **Post-MRI Reliability:** Research is needed to confirm the reliability of CGM sensors after exposure to MRI, addressing concerns about sensor functionality post-exposure.

- **Nursing Time and Motion Studies:** Evaluating the impact of CGM use on nursing workflow can help optimize protocols and improve efficiency in inpatient settings.
- **Cost-Effectiveness Analysis:** Comprehensive cost-effectiveness studies are necessary to justify the widespread adoption of CGMs in hospitals, balancing initial investment with long-term healthcare savings.

CGM Use in Pregnant Women:

- **Specialized Insulin Drip Protocols:** Laboring mothers with Type 1 or Type 2 diabetes may require specialized insulin drip protocols that necessitate hourly glucose monitoring.
- **Prenatal Approval:** Devices such as the Abbott FreeStyle Libre 2 and 3 are FDA-approved for prenatal use, providing continuous glucose monitoring for pregnant women.
- **Intrapartum Efficacy Studies:** Despite the extensive research on CGM use during pregnancy, more studies are needed to evaluate the efficacy of CGM use for insulin drip titration during the intrapartum period.

The adoption of CGM technology in the inpatient setting has shown considerable promise in improving patient outcomes through early identification and intervention of glycemic fluctuations. However, further research is required to address existing limitations, optimize technological integration, and establish cost-effective protocols. In particular, the use of CGMs in laboring mothers and the potential for CGM-assisted insulin drip titration during the intrapartum period present areas for future investigation.

Conclusion

Continuous Glucose Monitoring (CGM) has emerged as a game-changer in the management of diabetes, offering real-time insights into glucose levels and revolutionizing patient care.

The integration of CGM technology into outpatient diabetes care has ushered in a new era of personalized and proactive management. Recent studies have highlighted the superior efficacy of CGM compared to traditional fingerstick glucose monitoring, demonstrating improved glycemic control, reduced hypoglycemic events, and enhanced quality of life for patients.

CGM empowers patients to take control of their diabetes management by providing continuous and actionable data on glucose trends and patterns. Recent research has shown that CGM users experience greater satisfaction with their treatment regimen, increased adherence to medication and lifestyle modifications, and better long-term health outcomes compared to those using conventional monitoring methods.

Healthcare providers have also witnessed notable changes in outpatient diabetes care with the widespread adoption of CGM. Recent literature highlights the enhanced efficiency and accuracy of clinical decision-making enabled by CGM data, leading to more personalized treatment plans and improved patient-provider communication. Moreover, CGM facilitates remote monitoring and virtual consultations, allowing providers to deliver timely interventions and support to patients beyond traditional clinic settings.

The future of CGM in diabetes care holds immense promise for further innovation and advancement. Recent developments in CGM technology, including continuous glucose sensing, artificial intelligence algorithms, and interoperability with electronic health records, are poised to transform the delivery of diabetes care and improve patient outcomes. Future research should focus on addressing the remaining challenges and optimizing the integration of CGM into routine clinical practice. By leveraging recent findings and literature, healthcare providers can harness the full potential of CGM to revolutionize outpatient diabetes care, improve patient outcomes, and ultimately enhance the quality of life for individuals living with diabetes.

References

1. Castellana M, Parisi C, Di Molfetta S, et al. Efficacy and safety of flash glucose monitoring in patients with type 1 and type 2 diabetes: a systematic review and meta-analysis BMJ. Open Diabetes Res Care. 2020;8:e001092. https://doi.org/10.1136/bmjdrc-2019-001092.
2. Evans M, Welsh Z, Ells S, et al. The impact of flash glucose monitoring on glycaemic control as measured by HbA1c: a meta-analysis of clinical trials and real-world observational studies. Diabetes Ther. 2020;11:83–95. https://doi.org/10.1007/s13300-019-00720-0.
3. Nathanson D, Eeg-Olofsson K, Spelman T, et al. Retrospective controlled study shows intermittently-scanned CGM is associated with lower HbA1c and reduced hospitalisation for diabetes events in adults with T1DM in Sweden. In: Presented at EASD, 2-6 October 2023, Hamburg, Germany; 2023.
4. Forlenza GP, Kushner T, Messer LH, Wadwa RP, Sankaranarayanan S. Factory-calibrated continuous glucose monitoring: how and why it works, and the dangers of reuse beyond approved duration of wear. Diabetes Technol Ther. 2019;21(4):222–9. https://doi.org/10.1089/dia.2018.0401.
5. Lewis DM, Oser TK, Wheeler BJ. Continuous glucose monitoring. BMJ. 2023;380:e072420. https://doi.org/10.1136/bmj-2022-072420.
6. Leelarathna L, Evans ML, Neupane S, Rayman G, Lumley S, Cranston I, Narendran P, Barnard-Kelly K, Sutton CJ, Elliott RA, Taxiarchi VP, Gkountouras G, Burns M, Mubita W, Kanumilli N, Camm M, Thabit H, Wilmot EG, FLASH-UK Trial Study Group. Intermittently scanned continuous glucose monitoring for type 1 diabetes. N Engl J Med. 2022;387(16):1477–87. https://doi.org/10.1056/NEJMoa2205650.
7. Friedman JG, Cardona Matos Z, Szmuilowicz ED, Aleppo G. Use of continuous glucose monitors to manage type 1 diabetes mellitus: progress, challenges, and recommendations. Pharmgenomics Pers Med. 2023;16:263–76. https://doi.org/10.2147/PGPM.S374663.
8. Dexcom. n.d.. Retrieved from https://www.dexcom.com/en-us/g7-cgm-system.
9. Medtronic. n.d.. Retrieved from https://www.medtronicdiabetes.com/products/guardian-connect-continuous-glucose-monitoring-system.

10. Schierenbeck F, Franco-Cereceda A, Liska J. Accuracy of 2 different continuous glucose monitoring systems in patients undergoing cardiac surgery: intravascular microdialysis versus subcutaneous tissue monitoring. J Diabetes Sci Technol. 2017;11(1):108–16. https://doi.org/10.1177/1932296816651632.
11. Abbott. n.d.. FreeStyle Libre 3. Retrieved from https://www.freestyle.abbott/us-en/products/freestyle-libre-3.html.
12. Gavin JR, Bailey CJ. Real-world studies support use of continuous glucose monitoring in type 1 and type diabetes. Technol Ther. 2021;23:S3. S-19-S-27
13. Nathanson D, Svensson AM, Miftaraj M, Franzén S, Bolinder J, Eeg-Olofsson K. Effect of flash glucose monitoring in adults with type 1 diabetes: a nationwide, longitudinal observational study of 14,372 flash users compared with 7691 glucose sensor naive controls. Diabetologia. 2021;64(7):1595–603. https://doi.org/10.1007/s00125-021-05437-z.
14. Ascensia. (n.d.). Introducing the Eversense E3. Retrieved from https://www.ascensiadiabetes.com/eversense/.
15. Freckmann G, Pleus S, Grady M, Setford S, Levy B. Measures of accuracy for continuous glucose monitoring and blood glucose monitoring devices. J Diabetes Sci Technol. 2019;13(3):575–83. https://doi.org/10.1177/1932296818812062.
16. Pleus S, Stuhr A, Link M, Haug C, Freckmann G. Variation of mean absolute relative differences of continuous glucose monitoring systems throughout the day. J Diabetes Sci Technol. 2022;16(3):649–58. https://doi.org/10.1177/1932296821992373.
17. Edward R, Priefer R. A comparison of continuous glucose monitors (CGMs) in diabetes management: a systematic literature review. Primary Care Diabetes. 2023;17(6):529–34. https://doi.org/10.1016/j.pcd.2023.10.009.
18. Avari P, Lumb A, Flanagan D, et al. Continuous glucose monitoring within hospital: a scoping review and summary of guidelines from the Joint British Diabetes Societies for Inpatient Care. Journal of Diabetes Science and Technology. 2023;17(3):611–24. https://doi.org/10.1177/19322968221137338.
19. Spanakis EK, Cook CB, Kulasa K, et al. A consensus statement for continuous glucose monitoring metrics for inpatient clinical trials. J Diabetes Sci Technol. 2023;17(6):1527–52. https://doi.org/10.1177/19322968231191104.
20. Tripyla A, Herzig D, Joachim D, et al. Performance of a factory calibrated, real-time continuous glucose monitoring system during elective abdominal surgery. Diabetes Obes Metab. 2020;22(9):1678–82. https://doi.org/10.1111/dom.14073.
21. Thabit H, Prabhu JN, Mubita W, Fullwood C, Azmi S, Urwin A, Doughty I, Leelarathna L. Use of factory-calibrated real-time continuous glucose monitoring improves time in target and HbA1c in a multiethnic cohort of adolescents and young adults with type 1 diabetes: the MILLENNIALS Study. Diabetes Care. 2020;43(10):2537–43. https://doi.org/10.2337/dc20-0736.
22. Charleer S, De Block C, Van Huffel L, Broos B, Fieuws S, Nobels F, et al. Quality of life and glucose control after 1 year of nationwide reimbursement of intermittently scanned continuous glucose monitoring in adults living with type 1 diabetes (FUTURE): a prospective observational real-world cohort study. Diabetes Care. 2020;43:389–97. https://doi.org/10.2337/dc19-1610.
23. Finn E, Schlichting L, Grau L, Douglas IS, Pereira RI. Real-world accuracy of CGM in inpatient critical and noncritical care settings at a safety-net hospital. Diabetes Care. 2023;46(10):1825–30. https://doi.org/10.2337/dc23-0089.
24. McCall AL, Lieb DC, Gianchandani R, et al. Management of individuals with diabetes at high risk for hypoglycemia: an endocrine society clinical practice guideline. J Clin Endocrinol Metab. 2023;108:529.
25. Azhar A, Gillani SW, Mohiuddin G, Majeed RA. A systematic review on clinical implication of continuous glucose monitoring in diabetes management. J Pharmacy Bioallied Sci. 12020, 2(2):102–11. https://doi.org/10.4103/jpbs.JPBS_7_20.

26. Jacobs PG, Tyler NS, Vanderwerf SM, Mosquera-Lopez C, Seidl T, Cargill R, Branigan D, Ramsey K, Morris K, Benware S, Ward WK, Castle JR. Measuring glucose at the site of insulin delivery with a redox-mediated sensor. Biosens Bioelectron. 2020;165:112221. https://doi.org/10.1016/j.bios.2020.112221.
27. Guillot FH, Jacobs PG, Wilson LM, Youssef JE, Gabo VB, Branigan DL, Tyler NS, Ramsey K, Riddell MC, Castle JR. Accuracy of the Dexcom G6 Glucose Sensor during aerobic, resistance, and interval exercise in adults with type 1 diabetes. Biosensors (Basel). 2020;10(10):138. https://doi.org/10.3390/bios10100138.
28. Schaffer R. CGM as medicine technology benefits extend to type 2 diabetes. Endocrine today 2021, November.
29. American Diabetes Association Professional Practice Committee. 7. Diabetes Technology: Standards of Care in Diabetes—2024. Diabetes Care. 2024;47(Suppl. 1):S126–44. https://doi.org/10.2337/dc24-S007.
30. Dexcom. 2022. FDA grants breakthrough device designation for Dexcom hospital CGM system. Retrieved from https://investors.dexcom.com/news/news-details/2022/FDA-Grants-Breakthrough-Device-Designation-for-Dexcom-Hospital-CGM-System/default.aspx#:~:text=SAN%20DIEGO%2D%2D%20%28BUSINESS%20WIRE%29%2D%2DMar.%201%2C%202022%2D%2D%20DexCom%2C%20Inc.,for%20Dexcom%20CGM%20use%20in.
31. USFDA. 2023. MedWatch online voluntary reporting form. USFDA. Retrieved September 2, 2023, from https://www.accessdata.fda.gov/scripts/medwatch/index.cfm?action=reporting.home.
32. Dexcom. 2023. Dexcom. Retrieved December 20, 2023, from https://www.dexcom.com/en-us/hospitalfacts.
33. Korytkowski MT, Muniyappa R, Antinori-Lent K, Donihi AC, Drincic AT, Hirsch IB, Luger A, McDonnell ME, Murad MH, Nielsen C, Pegg C, Rushakoff RJ, Santesso N, Umpierrez GE. Management of hyperglycemia in hospitalized adult patients in non-critical care settings: an endocrine society clinical practice guideline. J Clin Endocrinol Metab. 2022;107(8):2101–28. https://doi.org/10.1210/clinem/dgac278.
34. Zelada H, Perez-Guzman MC, Chernavvsky DR, Galindo RJ. Continuous glucose monitoring for inpatient diabetes management: an update on current evidence and practice. Endocr Connect. 2023;12(10):e230180. https://doi.org/10.1530/EC-23-0180.
35. Perez-Guzman MC, Shang T, Zhang JY, Jornsay D, Klonoff DC. Continuous glucose monitoring in the hospital. Endocrinol Metab (Seoul). 2021;36(2):240–55. https://doi.org/10.3803/EnM.2021.201.
36. Oliver N. Diabetes Therapy podcast: real-world data for glucose sensing technologies in type 1 diabetes. Diabetes Ther. 2023;14:1–10. https://doi.org/10.1007/s13300-022-01331-y.
37. ElSayed NA, Aleppo G, Aroda VR, Bannuru RR, Brown FM, Bruemmer D, Collins BS, Hilliard ME, Isaacs D, Johnson EL, Kahan S, Khunti K, Leon J, Lyons SK, Perry ML, Prahalad P, Pratley RE, Seley JJ, Stanton RC, Gabbay RA, on behalf of the American Diabetes Association. 16. Diabetes Care in the Hospital: Standards of Care in Diabetes—2023. Diabetes Care. 2023;46(Suppl. 1):S267–78. https://doi.org/10.2337/dc23-S016.
38. Larkins MC, Thombare A. Point-of-care testing. [Updated 2023 May 29]. In: StatPearls. Treasure Island (FL): StatPearls Publishing; 2024. Available from: https://www.ncbi.nlm.nih.gov/books/NBK592387/.
39. Price CE, Fanelli JE, Aloi JA, Anzola SC, Vishneski SR, Saha AK, Woody CC, Segal S. Feasibility of intraoperative continuous glucose monitoring: an observational study in general surgery patients. J Clin Anesth. 2023;87:111090. https://doi.org/10.1016/j.jclinane.2023.111090.
40. Grunberger G, Sherr J, Allende M, Blevins T, Bode B, Handelsman Y, Hellman R, Lajara R, Roberts VL, Rodbard D, Stec C. American Association of Clinical Endocrinology clinical practice guideline: the use of advanced technology in the management of persons with diabetes mellitus. Endocrine Pract. 2021;27(6):505–37. https://doi.org/10.1016/j.eprac.2021.04.008.

41. Dogra P, Jialal I. Diabetic perioperative management [Updated 2022 Jun 19]. In: StatPearls. Treasure Island (FL): StatPearls Publishing; 2023. Available from: https://www.ncbi.nlm.nih.gov/books/NBK540965/.
42. Gianchandani R, Dubois E, Alexanian S, Rushakoff R. Preoperative, intraoperative, and postoperative glucose management. In: Drasnin B, editor. Managing diabetes and hyperglycemia in the hospital setting. Alexandria, VA: American Diabetes Association; 2016. p. 129–44.
43. Heinemann L, Schoemaker M, Schmelzeisen-Redecker G, et al. Benefits and limitations of MARD as a performance parameter for continuous glucose monitoring in the interstitial space. J Diabetes Sci Technol. 2020;14(1):135–50. https://doi.org/10.1177/1932296819855670.
44. Aggarwal A, Pathak S, Goyal R. Clinical and economic outcomes of continuous glucose monitoring system (CGMS) in patients with diabetes mellitus: a systematic literature review. Diabetes Res Clin Pract. 2022;186:109825. https://doi.org/10.1016/j.diabres.2022.109825.
45. American Diabetes Association Professional Practice Committee. 16. Diabetes Care in the hospital: standards of care in diabetes—2024. Diabetes Care. 2024;47(Suppl. 1):S295–306. https://doi.org/10.2337/dc24-S016.
46. Carlsson CJ, Nørgaard K, Oxbøll AB, Søgaard MIV, Achiam MP, Jørgensen LN, Eiberg JP, Palm H, Sørensen HBD, Meyhof CS, Aasvang EK. Continuous glucose monitoring reveals perioperative hypoglycemia in most patients with diabetes undergoing major surgery: a prospective cohort study. Ann Surg. 2023;277(4):603–11. https://doi.org/10.1097/SLA.0000000000005246.
47. Michel M, Lucke-Wold B. Diabetes management in spinal surgery. J Clin Images Med Case Rep. 2022;3(6):1906.
48. Sreedharan R, Khanna S, Shaw A. Perioperative glycemic management in adults presenting for elective cardiac and non-cardiac surgery. Perioper Med. 2023;12:13. https://doi.org/10.1186/s13741-023-00302-6.
49. Rajan N, Duggan EW, Abdelmalak BB, Butz S, Rodriguez LV, Vann MA, Joshi GP. Society for ambulatory anesthesia updated consensus statement on perioperative blood glucose management in adult patients with diabetes mellitus undergoing ambulatory surgery. Anesth Analg. 2024; https://doi.org/10.1213/ANE.0000000000006791.
50. Pinson K, Kim J, Gottesman B, Stanley V, Sharma N, Kobayashi E, Majithia A, Ramos GA. Glycemic control in labor: Comparing time in ange (TIR) among gravidas with and without pre-gestational diabetes. Glycemic control in labor: comparing time in range (TIR) among gravidas with and without pre-gestational diabetes. Am J Obstet Gynecol. 2024;230(1):S419. https://doi.org/10.1016/j.ajog.2023.11.812.
51. Lai M, Weng J, Yang J, Gong Y, Fang F, Li N, Kang M, Xu X, Wang Y. Effect of continuous glucose monitoring compared with self-monitoring of blood glucose in gestational diabetes patients with HbA1c < 6%: a randomized controlled trial. Front Endocrinol (Lausanne). 2023;14:1174239. https://doi.org/10.3389/fendo.2023.1174239.
52. Murphy HR. Roadmap to the effective use of continuous glucose monitoring in pregnancy. Diabetes Spectr. 2023;36(4):315–9. https://doi.org/10.2337/dsi23-0004.
53. Tauschmann M, Forlenza G, Hood K, et al. ISPAD Clinical Practice Consensus Guidelines 2022: diabetes technologies: glucose monitoring. Pediatr Diabetes. 2022;23(8):1390–405. https://doi.org/10.1111/pedi.13451.
54. Charleer S, Gillard P, Vandoorne E, Cammaerts K, Mathieu C, Casteels K. Intermittently scanned continuous glucose monitoring is associated with high satisfaction but increased HbA1c and weight in well-controlled youth with type 1 diabetes. Pediatric Diabetes. 2020;21:1465–74. https://doi.org/10.1111/pedi.13128.
55. Crossen S, Xing G, Hoch JS. Changing costs of type 1 diabetes care among US children and adolescents. Pediatr Diabetes. 2020;21:644–8. https://doi.org/10.1111/pedi.12996.
56. Dexcom. 2023. Display device screens. Dexcom. Retrieved June 2023, from display device screens.

57. Tamborlane WV, Beck RW, Bode BW, et al. Juvenile Diabetes Research Foundation Continuous Glucose Monitoring Study Group. Continuous glucose monitoring and intensive treatment of type 1 diabetes. N Engl J Med. 2008;359:1464–76.
58. Tumminia A, Crimi S, Sciacca L, et al. Efficacy of real-time continuous glucose monitoring on glycaemic control and glucose variability in type 1 diabetic patients treated with either insulin pumps or multiple insulin injection therapy: a randomized controlled crossover trial. Diabetes Metab Res Rev. 2015;31:61–8. 32. Hansen KW, Bibby BM. The frequency of intermittently scanned glucose and diurnal variation of glycemic metrics. J Diabetes Sci Technol. 27 May 2021 [Epub ahead of print]. DOI: 10.1177/19322968211019382
59. Urakami T, Yoshida K, Kuwabara R, et al. Frequent scanning using flash glucose monitoring contributes to better glycemic control in children and adolescents with type 1 diabetes. J Diabetes Investig. 2021; https://doi.org/10.1111/jdi.13618.
60. Hohendorff J, Gumprecht J, Mysliwiec M, Zozulinska-Ziolkiewicz D, Malecki MT. Intermittently scanned continuous glucose monitoring data of Polish patients from real-life conditions: more scanning and better glycemic control compared to worldwide data. Diabetes Technol Ther. 2021;23:577–85.
61. Aleppo G, Ruedy KJ, Riddlesworth TD, et al. REPLACE-BG Study Group. REPLACE-BG: a randomized trial comparing continuous glucose monitoring with and without routine blood glucose monitoring in adults with well-controlled type 1 diabetes. Diabetes Care. 2017;40:538–45.
62. U.S. Food and Drug Administration. FDA News Release: FDA approves first continuous glucose monitoring system for adults not requiring blood sample calibration; 2017. Available from https://www.fda.gov/NewsEvents/Newsroom/PressAnnouncements/ucm577890.htm.
63. Lameijer A, Lommerde N, Dunn TC, et al. Flash glucose monitoring in the Netherlands: increased monitoring frequency is associated with improvement of glycemic parameters. Diabetes Res Clin Pract. 2021;177:108897.
64. U.S. Food and Drug Administration. FDA News Release: FDA expands indication for continuous glucose monitoring system, first to replace fingerstick testing for diabetes treatment decisions, 2016. Available from https://www.fda.gov/newsevents/newsroom/pressannouncements/ucm534056.htm.

Chapter 4
Basic Principles of Automated Insulin Delivery Systems

Eden Miller

For several individuals living with diabetes, insulin is a life sustaining and necessary hormone to control dysfunctional glycemia. For those with type 1 diabetes, insulin is a life-sustaining hormone, and must replace it externally to maintain normal metabolism. For individuals with type 2 diabetes, insulin is often initiated using long-acting or basal insulin to provide a foundation for glucose control. As their disease progresses, many type 2's will be required to add rapid or bolus insulin to cover mealtime and other metabolic needs. In contrast, type 1 diabetes by nature of its immune destruction of the beta cell necessitates a complete replacement of insulin at a physiologic level.

Over the years, the delivery of this insulin into the body has evolved. The very first insulin administration over 100 years ago was injected using a glass reusable syringe with an 18-gauge needles requiring frequent sharpening using stones [1]. These were fragile and a daily painful experience. A few decades later, they were replaced with disposable plastic syringes, marked with varying units, and capped with smaller gauge, shorter needles. These advancements dramatically lessened the burden of insulin administration. Further convenience of prefilled pens with U100/ml and concentrated U200/ml, U300/ml, and U500/ml insulin helped overcome the barriers of volume, dosing, and improved portability. They are capable of 5–2-unit delivery, capped with pen needles as small as 33 G and 4 mm in length. These devices allow for increased portability, privacy, and ease of use for insulin injections. More recently, manual and spring-driven patch delivery systems provided users to wear their insulin allowing for delivery of bolus or both basal and bolus

E. Miller (✉)
Diabetes Nation, Diabetes and Obesity Care, Bend, OR, USA

Adjunct Faculty University Health Sciences Pomona, Pomona, CA, USA

Adjunct Faculty COMP NW Medical School Lebanon, Lebanon, OR, USA
e-mail: eden@diabetesandobesity-care.com

S. Fishman (ed.), *Advances in Diabetes Technology*, Contemporary Endocrinology, https://doi.org/10.1007/978-3-031-75352-7_4

insulin. Rising out of this administration history are the continuous subcutaneous insulin infusion (CSII) or also known as insulin pumps. Their development has radically changed the diabetes insulin management landscape. This chapter will discuss these devices, their history, development, integration of continuous glucose monitoring, and dosing algorithms to provide a near physiologic external pancreas.

The very first prototype of the insulin pump was created by Dr. Arnold Kadish in 1963. Initially, this system was large, worn on the back, cumbersome, and required intravenous insulin delivery. From there Dr. Ernst Friedrich Pfeiffer in 1974 combined IV continuous glucose monitoring and insulin infusion with the first closed-loop system called "Biostator. " [2] His creation, though rudimentary, provided the foundation for future advancement and the feasibility of a closed-loop system. Wearable insulin pumps were available in 1976, by Dean Kamen. The first version was termed the "blue brick" and later the "auto syringe." Despite this burdensome therapy, it did mark the beginning of technology as a tool to assist in insulin delivery and would pave the way for ultimate external automated pancreas. Out of these evolved systems more compact and lighter weight. Delivery features started with basal then expanded to mealtime and correction bolus. A new vocabulary was created to define the features. Shortly after in 1979, Al Mann with Pacesetter systems became interested in developing a more user-friendly smaller insulin pump. His first study participant in early 1980 was Freddi Fredrickson. She was a diabetes nurse educator with type 1 diabetes who went on this pump as a study participant to determine the long-term risk and benefits to this new technology. Later in her career, she teamed up with MiniMed, becoming the pump company's seventh employee. For 24 years, she contributed to the development of insulin delivery devices, even working alongside Al Mann, an innovator in the field. To date, she has been the longest user of an insulin delivery device, all the while continuing to call for insulin pumps to become the standard of care in the treatment of diabetes. This dream of hers continues to push this standard forward, and prescribers are now seeing the utility of insulin delivery devices, starting to overcome the educational barrier to full implementation. However, it as a Japanese group led by Motoaki Shichir in early 1980 that created the first wearable subcutaneous artificial pancreas. Small enough to be place in a pocket, is consisted of a sensor, microcomputer, and two roller pumps that delivered both insulin and glucagon under the skin or subcutaneously in contrast to the Biostator which was delivered intravenously.

MiniMed in 1983 made available their first commercial pump the MiniMed 502, and since then several versions further enhance the features and experience to the utilizer while improving physiologic insulin replacement. It was 1986 when MiniMed released the first implantable insulin pump to deliver intraperitoneally termed continuous intraperitoneal insulin infusion (CIPII). . One advantage of this system is that insulin is delivered directly into the portal system which mimics normal body physiology as the pancreas and hepatic system are connected in a similar manner. The insulin delivered through this device allowed for rapid absorption and a quicker physiologic insulin action. Current external pumps still are challenged by getting the insulin in fast enough through the subcutaneous tissue. Studies demonstrated that users of this system with type 1 diabetes had tight glucose control with low variability and less hypoglycemia. In 2000, the MiniMed (MIP 2001) version with a longer battery life and improved software was released, but because of catheter occlusion and under delivery of insulin, the future of peritoneal insulin pumps was coming to an end. These systems required complex surgical application and despite their near-physiologic insulin control these systems were utilized less and less. As newer more reliable external pumps were being developed a shift from the implantable systems to the external pumps began. Official they were discontinued in 2007 as in 2003 the MiniMed Paradigm 512 system was released. The Paradigm 512 system was termed a "smart pump" as it could display the co-developed BD Link® blood glucose meter. This self-monitoring blood glucose monitor wirelessly imported the readings from the meter to the MiniMed pump, using that information with the onboard Bolus Wizard Calculator programmed by the health care provider, it would suggest insulin dose based on the glucose level and preprogrammed information of insulin to carbohydrate ratio and insulin correction factor. This system would provide the suggested calculation to the wearer to administer manually. Medtronic went on from there in 2006 to develop the MiniMed Paradigm Real-Time system. It marked the first integrated insulin pump and continuous glucose monitor that were both developed by Medtronic to be used in this new system which was a steppingstone to the development of automated insulin delivery systems (AIDS) . By utilizing continuous glucose sensors to provide data to the programmed insulin delivery device the integration of these two distinct technology platforms allowed for partial "closed-loop" system. The partial is when basal rate adjustments and insulin suspension are determined from real-time continuous glucose monitoring information. It allows for the wearer to have more automated control with less individual engagement. Hybrid closed looping is another term, and this can refer to more advanced continuous glucose monitoring with predictive decision-making such as correction blousing, basal rate augmentation, and hypoglycemic prevention. In 2009, Medtronic launched the MiniMed Veo System, with a Low Glucose Suspend feature that automatically halts insulin delivery when sensor glucose levels hit a preset low threshold. MiniMed 530G with an Enlite sensor has been recognized as a first-generation artificial pancreas device system with threshold suspend development of a real-time continuous glucose sensor-augmented insulin pump deliver was the necessary step toward the future development of a fully "closed-loop" insulin delivery system or an artificial pancreas (AP). This device was approved by the FDA in 2013 for the use of diabetes patients >16 years of age. Then Medtronic introduced the MiniMed 640G system in 2015, taking one step closer to the artificial pancreas system. This system has integrated smart features such as active insulin tracking, a bolus progress bar, and enhanced battery life. In 2017, the first hybrid closed-loop system, the MiniMed 670G insulin pump with a Guardian 3 sensor, was licensed by the FDA for T1D therapy of children 7 years and older. When in auto mode, it functions as a hybrid closed-loop system that automatically controls basal insulin delivery every 5 min based on the CGM values to hold BG levels tightly to the specific target of 70–180 or specified by the prescriber. Today the Medtronic 780 G with Guardian 4 sensor continues to advance insulin infusion with extended infusion set wear time, auto correction basal and bolus, and "meal detection" technology.

Another option entered the market with the Animus IR 1200 insulin pump. It was more compact, about the size of a pager and provided utilizers programmable hourly basal rates, insulin duration (insulin on board), safety alarms and insulin mealtime calculator and extended bolus delivery options to cover longer mealtimes, and higher fat foods that often extend the glycemic affect. In 2005, Johnson and Johnson purchased the Animus group but later left the insulin delivery device arena, in part due to the lack of utilization of their system and rapid expanding technology options being developed but other companies. They formally discontinued the Animus production and support in 2017.

Yet another pump was developed, but this version was back to the intraperitoneal deliver of insulin by Accu-Chek® Diaport system (Roche Diabetes Care) the MIP 2007C. There was a percutaneous port attached to an external pump such as the is implanted beneath the subcutaneous tissue in the lower abdomen, this subcutaneous port has a catheter that is inserted just into the peritoneum and directed toward the liver. After implantation, the pump reservoir is refilled by an outpatient health care provider with concentrated insulin at least every 3 months. The Accu-Chek® Diaport system enables infusion of insulin into the peritoneal cavity through an Accu-Chek insulin pump and an infusion set. Historically Continuous Intraperitoneal Insulin Infusion (CIPII) has been shown as a quit effective treatment option for persons with T1D diabetes. However, their are barriers to CIPII, include higher cost of an invasive surgical procedure, cannula blockage, peritoneal infection, and thrombosis of the portal-vein. As a result, this treatment option has been replaced as the standard of care and is exceeding rare to be considered or even in use.

A similar fate was seen in the Roche pump subcutaneous insulin delivery system that was introduced in 2012. It was paired with the Accu-Chek meter to display glucose data and provided similar features as the Animus but ongoing occlusion errors and lack of utilization in the US market ended it short run in 2017 [3].

The limitations of the tethered pumps (IDD with tubed infusion sites) led to the development of "patch pumps": pumps that are free of infusion sets, small, lightweight, and attached to the skin through an adhesive. These on body tubeless pumps are loaded with maximum of 220 units. Patch pumps offer additional comfort and flexibility to users, especially children, those that are active, or occupations pose tubing hazards and pull out. In 2011, Insulet introduced Omnipod, the first tubeless insulin pump. It comprises an integrated infusion set within the pod, and automated inserter that converses wirelessly with an integrated personal diabetes manager (PDM) . The Omnipod patch pump allows complete freedom to the users to engage in routine activities without tubing [4].

There are also two on body patch insulin delivery systems that are not considered pumps as they are manually operated, or spring driven. These such devices are the V-Go (Mankind) and the CeQur Simplicity (CeQur Corporation). simplified patch insulin delivery models became available on the market in 2010 and 2022, respectively. The V-Go delivers 24 h of rapid acting insulin with three available hourly basal rates using an engineered non-mechanical design, and it allows for on demand 2-unit increment of bolus administrations. The CeQur is an on body manually insulin delivering device that provided bolus insulin in 2-unit increments, holds 200 units, and can be used for up to 3 days.

Insulin Pump Therapy in Clinical Practice

Now that the brief history foundation of insulin pump has be set, it is time to begin the process of identifying, prescribing, and initiating insulin pump therapy with or without continuous glucose monitoring. Remember to match the pump to the person, choosing the features, connectivity and accessibility based on the patient's needs. The administration of insulin through mechanical means is not necessarily the end goal for person with diabetes, rather it is attempting to mimic pancreatic physiology through an automated insulin delivery systems or (AIDS) using integrated continuous glucose management when this system would better serve the patients insulin management needs. These integrated diabetes-related technology devices can provide an external pancreas that monitors, administers, titrates, and suspends insulin while predicting glucose patterns using an algorithm capable of learning the metabolic nuances of the wearer.

With this expansion of insulin delivery, a whole new pump language or terminology has come about. An understanding of this terminology will equip prescribers to begin the process of initiating pump use in their practice settings. The first term, *basal rate*, is the programmable hourly insulin rate that addresses the circadian rhythm hormonal effects and changes in daily activities that impact glucose control in a 24-h day. The programmable basal rate allows for customization on an hour-by-hour basis according to these individualized daily needs. This replaces the long-acting injection used for patients on the basal bolus regimen. *Bolus* insulin administration for meals has morphed from fixed dosing to calculation based on insulin to carbohydrate ratios. *Correction boluses* and *insulin sensitivity factors* became a new metric further customizing insulin delivery. Advanced features such as *dual wave, square wave*, and/or *extended boluses* allowed for meals with varying nutritional content such as high fat or longer duration of meal. *Insulin duration* or more specifically the length of insulin active in the individually metabolically became known as *insulin on board* to allow for reverse calculation to further fine-tune recommended mealtime and correction insulin boluses. The dawn of continuous glucose monitoring provided the missing piece to begin development of external systems capable of delivering a physiologic insulin experience. Once CGM accuracy increased to a level to allow for insulin decision-making, these symptoms became paired, and the introduction of automation began. Safety was first on the list of pump to do's, allowing CGM data to provide a low glycemic threshold for insulin administration suspension, thus decreasing the risk of hypoglycemia. Systems improved to allow for reinitiating of insulin administration once glucose rose above hypoglycemic threshold. From there CGM predictive algorithms allowing for basal rate alterations to address hyperglycemia and hypoglycemia events. This marked a point in development termed partial hybrid closed-loop insulin pump. Manufacturers improved upon the predictive algorithm recommendations as CGM accuracy improved and lack of sensor calibration required with some CGM systems. Most recently, a completely automated insulin delivery system allows for wearers glycemic control using a full auto mode algorithm controlling for hyperglycemia, increased time in range (TIR), improved avoidance of hypoglycemia, and adaptations of the pump by learning the patterns of the person over time and adjusting the delivery setting based on the information through the CGM. The user only needs to calculate and enter carbohydrates, continuously wear an integrated sensor, and the rest is done by the pump. This marks the beginning of the first artificial external pancreas, with a future of fine tuning and customization to come.

Now that we have had an overview, let's take a deeper dive going beyond terminology and into prescribing in clinical practice. We start by answering the question of which persons with diabetes should pump? I get this question most often and the person with diabetes is always at the center of my response. A person should consider an insulin delivery device (IDD) when the current therapeutic glycemic intervention is unable to meet their needs both physically and emotionally [5]. A pump is not advised to make diabetes easier for the person, even though it often can, but rather the individual desires an expanded way of administering insulin that can also overcome the barriers and distress in diabetes. Secondly, you always match the patient to the pump, not the other way around. That is why familiarity or at least directional knowledge of the different systems available will assist in pairing the best pump to the person. Two such resources are online sites Diabeteswise.org and Diabeteswisepro.org. The first is a comprehensive patient facing site the walks the user through all forms of diabetes technology; CMG, IDD, and connected insulin pens, providing the user nonbranded information in all areas to assist in the decision-making process. Equally as beneficial the corresponding professional site, walks health care providers through the various options and assists in ordering and coverage determination. Finally, there exists several educational tools regarding IDD and sensors that can be found at the American Diabetes Association, *www.diabetes.org*, and American Association of Diabetes Educators website *www.diabeteseducator.org* to name a few.

Once the pump option has been chosen for the individual, then coverage determination and approval are needed. In the past, there were limited options for IDD and coverage would often determine the patient choice. However, today we see that less of an issue, but it is not a guarantee. So be mindful, some insurance plans provide only one pump option which does not allow for patient selection. In some instances, appeal can be made if a particular pump feature is needed for the individual. This will require additional documentation of the medical necessity for the specific insulin pump desired. As a generality, pumps are covered for most persons with have autoimmune positive type 1 diabetes with Medicaid, Commercial and Medicare plans. These individuals are considered insulin absent, and pumping repeatedly has been shown to improved control, quality of life, and acute complications. Commercially insured type 2 diabetes persons on multiple daily injections lacking glycemic control or possessing complications such as CKD, CAD, or acute diabetes-related events like hypo- and hyperglycemic requiring advance medication attention will be eligible for insulin pumps. For those with type 2 DM with Medicare on multiple daily injections who become deficient in the amount of native insulin produced; morning C-peptide less than 2.0 with serum glucose less than 200 mg/dl at the time of the draw will qualify for consideration for insulin pump approval. Medicaid coverage of IDD for persons with type 2 DM varies by plan and by state. These generalities should not dissuade you from considering insulin pump therapies for your patients. If you do not try at all for acquisition or coverage, it is 100% not going to be obtained. I cannot stress enough to match the IDD to the person. Coverage and prescriber familiarity with these devices is essential but should not be the driving factor for selection. Consider the pump features, level of engagement and comprehension of that person, and ultimately what do they need the pump to do for them.

In the table below (Fig. 4.1), you can see an overview of the advancements in glucose monitoring technology (CGM) that allows monitoring of glucose levels every 1–5 min, real-time alerts for hypoglycemic/hyperglycemic events, integration with IDD (pumps), and glucose data for calculations for AID (automatic insulin delivery) CGM paired pumps. CGM devices are continually advancing in accuracy, size, interoperability, and length of wear. These systems will become the standard for glucose monitoring and finger sticking will fade into the past.

Prior to onboarding of any insulin delivery device, there are individualized settings that need to be calculated and determined. These can be done by the prescriber or sent as an order to the CDCES pump educator.

The first such calculation is the *total insulin requirement*. This is the total amount of insulin required to cover the 24-h day, including basal, bolus for food, and correction for glucose levels not at target. There are several ways to estimate this

FDA-Approved Personal CGM Devices

	Abbott FreeStyle Libre 14-day/2/3	Dexcom G6 G7 approved by FDA 12/8	Medtronic Guardian Sensor 3 (pump integrated) and Guardian Connect (stand-alone)	Senseonics Eversense
Approved labeling	Replaces fingersticks for treatment decisions; no fingerstick calibration required	Replaces fingersticks for treatment decisions; no fingerstick calibration required	Requires ≥2 fingerstick calibrations/d	Replaces fingersticks for treatment decisions; requires ≥2 fingerstick calibrations/d
Age	≥18 y/≥4 y/≥4 y	≥2 y	≥14y	≥18 y
Medicare coverage	Yes/Yes/Not Yet	Yes	Sensor 3: Yes; Connect: No	Yes
Wear length	14 d	10 d	7 d	90/180 d 360 day
Warm-up	1 hr	2 hr/27 min	2 hr	24 hours after implementation
Alarms	No/Yes/Yes	Yes	Yes	Yes
Data Display/ Integration	Reader; Android and iPhone Apps	Reader; Android and iPhone Apps; smartwatches; Tandem t:slim X2 pump.	Reader; Android and iPhone Apps; 630G, 670G or 770G pump; Guardian Connect	Android and iPhone Apps
Form	Disposable transmitter integrated with sensor patch	G6: Transmitter (3-month use) separate from sensor/G7 integrated	Transmitter (rechargeable) separate from sensor	Transmitter (rechargeable) separate from sensor
Accuracy* (lower numbers are more accurate)	11.4%/9.3%/7.9%[1]	9%/8.2%[1]	9.6%/9-11%[1]	8.5%-9.5%[1]
Expense[2]	Least expensive	2nd most expense	2nd least expensive	Most expensive

*Accuracy measured by MARD (mean absolute relative difference) relative to **VENOUS** glucose. Lower numbers indicate a more accurate device.

[1]Accuracy figures provided by manufacturers.
[2]What is a CGM and how do I choose one? Healthline Diabetes Mine. Updated December 14, 2021. Accessed February 12, 2023. https://www.healthline.com/diabetesmine/ what-is-continuous-glucose-monitor-and-choosing-one

Fig. 4.1 Graphic created by Dr. Eden Miller

number, and it will provide a foundation to build upon with initiating and programming insulin delivery devices.

There are several ways to determine total daily insulin requirement and to follow are a few examples of how to calculate this for everyone. Approximately 40–50% of the total daily insulin dose is to replace insulin overnight, when you are fasting and between meals. This is called background or basal insulin replacement. I explain to patients the basal rate is the like the idle on your car, it keeps the engine running but isn't enough to cover food and increased insulin needs. The basal or background insulin dose usually within a consistent daily range but can vary hour by hour. The remaining 50–60% of the total daily insulin dose is for carbohydrate coverage (food) and high blood sugar correction. This is called the bolus insulin replacement.

The general calculation for the body's daily insulin requirement in pounds is as follows:

$$\text{Total Daily Insulin Requirement}\left(\text{in units of insulin}\right) = \text{Weight in Pounds} \div 4$$

If using body weight in kilograms:

$$\text{Total daily insulin requirement}\left(\text{in units of insulin}\right) = 0.55 \times \text{total weight in kilograms}$$

If the individual is currently utilizing basal insulin plus bolus insulin you simply total up the amount used in a typical 24-h day.

Now you have one of the foundational settings, total daily dose, to begin calculating insulin requirements to be programmed into the insulin delivery device.

Let's now explore how to calculate the basal or hourly infusion rate of insulin for the 24-h day. This basal rate will provide the wearer an hourly programmed infusion rate of insulin using analog or rapid-acting insulin. Since insulin infusion will be delivered continuously through a pump to provide for the patients' basal metabolic needs, long-acting basal insulin is no longer necessary. This rate can be calculated using the following formulas.

Using the estimated total daily insulin dose, multiply that number by .4 or .5 this is your total daily basal dose. Then divide by 24 h which gives you the unit per hour basal rate.

Here is an example for an individual with type 2 diabetes.

Lets consider a 220-pound (100 kg) male with type 2 DM transitioning to an insulin delivery device. The TDD is calculated using the formula weight in pounds; 220 ÷ 4 would be a total daily dose of 55 units. Then multiplying that number by .4 (less aggressive basal) or .5 (more aggressive basal) which would be the estimated basal requirements = to 22–27.5 units. Then divide that number by 24 h and you now have the estimated hourly basal rate to be programmed into the pump. Some individual could have one fixed basal rate per hour for the entire 24-h period or others may require customized time segments basal rates based on diurnal insulin needs and sensitivity. Generally, more insulin is required in the early am due to diurnal levels of growth and cortisol, adjustments based on metabolic needs, activities of daily living, or reduction of hypoglycemia such as in the fasting overnight hours. Less variable type 2 DM individuals may have the same basal rate for the 24-h time period, or adjustments based on hormonal insulin sensitivity pattern such as 12–6 am the basal rate is lowered to minimize risk of hypoglycemia, higher in early day from 6 am–12 pm, lower in the afternoon 12 pm–5 pm due to increased insulin sensitivity and activity, and slightly higher from 5 pm to 12 am (midnight) due to increased feeding and less movement.

Calculating basal insulin for those with type 1 DM is similar but as they are more insulin sensitive, the weight in pounds divided by .3–.5 units with time interval adjustment due to effects of diurnal hormones. Often a dynamic basal program is needed to accommodate the daily fluctuating insulin needs rather than static basal rate, taking into account the activity level, lifestyle, and hormonal effects throughout the 24 day.

For pediatric type 1 DM, insulin doses with newly diagnosed type 1 diabetes vary widely from 0.2 units/kg/day to 0.8 units/kg/day. Generally, if this is a new onset type 1 pediatric patient you should be more conservative utilizing the lower calculated amount as they are often in the honeymoon period of the disease. From there adjustments could be determined based on further analysis of the glucose data and response to insulin.

Another method of basal calculation uses the total dose a long-acting injectable basal insulin the individual is injecting and dividing that number by 24 h. Some practitioners multiply this number by .8 since using analog rapid-acting insulin is more metabolically active and often requires fewer total units to provide basal coverage. Of note, when long-acting basal insulin doses exceed .5 units per kg/day per or >100 units daily the mathematically calculation starts to break down. If this is the case, return to the weight-based calculation to better estimate total daily dose and basal needs.

Now that we have determined the total daily dose and basal rate, the insulin correction factor, or amount of insulin to reach the targeted glucose range can be determined using the following formulas.

$$\begin{aligned} \textit{Correction Factor} &= 1800 \div \text{Total Daily Insulin Dose} \\ &= 1\,\text{unit of insulin will reduce the blood sugar so many mg / dl.} \\ &\quad \text{This calculation is termed the Rule of "1800".} \end{aligned}$$

Let's do an example:

- Assume your total daily insulin dose (TDI) =220 lbs. ÷ 4 = 55 units

In this example, the correction factor would be determined by taking 1800 ÷ TDI (55 units) = 1 unit insulin will drop reduce the blood sugar level by 33 mg/dl. While the calculation is 1 unit will drop the blood sugar 33 mg/dl, to make it easier most people will round up or round down the number so the suggested correction factor may be 1 unit of rapid acting insulin will drop the blood sugar about 35 mg/dl. This correction factor will be entered into the IDD and provide the calculations for insulin required to reach target during mealtimes or episodes of hyperglycemia.

Insulin to Carbohydrate Ratio (ICR)

The calculation of *mealtime bolus* insulin is the amount needed to cover the effects of food on the glucose. The insulin to carbohydrate ratio (ICR) equals how many grams of carbohydrate are covered by 1 unit of insulin to get maintain glucose control from premeal to end of meal at about 2–4 h afterwards. This number can be calculated based on insulin per grams of carbohydrate or insulin per carbohydrate exchange which has a base of 1 exchange equal to 15 g of carbohydrate. This calculation rule can be the same for each meal breakfast lunch and dinner or can be different by the time of day or size of meal. There is a diurnal or hormonal effect of the glycemia day where most persons require more insulin or a more aggressive ratio for breakfast, least for lunch and second most for dinner, but this could vary based on timing of meal, amount of food, and individual variability. This calculation can be made using weight based, generalized starting point based on type of diabetes and age of individual or trial and error.

This can be calculated using the Rule of "500": Carbohydrate Bolus Calculation

Weight-based insulin bolus calculation is done by the carbohydrate coverage ratio: 500 ÷ Total Daily Insulin Dose = 1 unit insulin covers so the calculated grams of carbohydrate.

As a starting point, one unit of rapid-acting insulin will dispose of 15 g of carbohydrate for those with type 2 diabetes, and 1 per 30 g of carb for individuals with type 1. Young Pediatric patients' recommendation is to start at .5–1 unit per 30 g of carbohydrate. One way to help determine this "rule" or calculation is to have the individual ingest a known number of grams of carbohydrate. Take the starting premeal glucose, apply the ICR estimation to the carbohydrate meal that is eaten completely within a short period of time, administer the calculated insulin (do not add additional insulin to correct for hyperglycemia during this exercise) using rapid-acting analog insulin and recheck the glucose level following the meal at least 2 h. It may take up to 3 or generally at most 4 h for the insulin to have its full effect as each person's insulin duration varies. In addition, if using regular insulin, the time duration can be even longer at 5 or more hours. The post meal or end of insulin duration glucose is measured. If the pre- and post meal glucose are near each other, <25 points variation then the ICR used is confirmed. If the post meal glucose is lower than the premeal, then consider increasing the carbs to insulin ratio to avoid hypoglycemia. Conversely if the post meal glucose is elevated beyond the premeal glucose the carbohydrates need to be lowered that is covered by one unit of insulin. Another trick that I use in clinical practice is to take the variation in the premeal and post meal glucose subtract those numbers and divide by the insulin sensitivity factor or correction factor the amount that is left is the additional units needed to add or subtracted from the initial ICR.

Another way to calculate the carbohydrate coverage ratio is to do the following calculation = 500 ÷ TDI (40 units) but this assumes you know the total daily insulin from basal bolus calculations = 1unit insulin/12 g CHO

This example above assumes that you have a consistent response to insulin throughout the day with each meal.

Let's try another example. A person with type 2 DM is going to ingest a known carbohydrate meal of 45 g, their premeal glucose is 150. Using the 1 per 15 g of carb (ICR) calculation we estimate 3 units for the meal, and it is administered right at or 15 min prior to the meal. The person then checks their glucose 2–2.5 h post meal. They report their glucose is 225 m/dl. You subtract 225–150 and get 75. Then using their insulin sensitivity factor or correction factor of 1 per 25 above target of 150 you divide 75 (deficit) by 25 (ISF) and get 3 units needed to correct to target. Then take the units given which were 3 plus the additional 3 needed for a total of 6 units for that 45-g carbohydrate meal. Dividing the 45 g of carb by 6 units equals 7.5 which meals a rule of 1 unit per 7.5 g of carb could be this individual's insulin to carbohydrate ratio. You can see there are a few methods of how to estimate or calculate this for the individual. This recommendation is an educated guess and confirmation with ongoing follow-up with the individual is necessary. These insulin to carbohydrate rations can vary from 4–45 g or more of carbohydrate per unit depending on an individual's sensitivity to insulin, age, and type of diabetes. In addition, insulin sensitivity can also vary according to the time of day as insulin resistance is greatest in the am least in the afternoon and second greatest in evening often do to meal size and fat content. So, a person may have one insulin to carbohydrate ratio for breakfast and different ones for lunch or dinner. Their breakfast insulin-to-carbohydrate ratio might be breakfast 1:8 g, lunch 1:15 g, and dinner 1:12 g.

Finally, the ICR can also be affected by physical activity, stress level, illness, and fat content of meal ingested, and this higher level learning will come with time, as the prescriber and person journey together.

Now let's discuss some special bolus deliveries. The *square wave, extended wave, or dual wave bolus* are features available with some pumps to allow for a bolus insulin to be dosed incrementally administered over a time period, rather than all at once. One could say this sounds like a temporary basal; however, basal rates don't tend to approach bolus rates which could be 3 to 5 times higher. This feature is utilized when meals are extended over a long period of time, social events, or types of food with higher fat content or delayed absorption of the carbohydrate occurs and the timing of the food an insulin has the potential to be mismatched. The square wave bolus or another terminology is 100% extended bolus is given over a pre-determined time period. An example could be a person is anticipating consuming a particular amount of carbohydrate of an extended period such as a dinner party. Let's say they are going to eat 60 g of carb and their insulin to carbohydrate ratio is 1 per 15 g of carb so 4 units are required to cover the meal, but that meal will be consumed over an hour. The bolus could be delivered over an hour but square wave or extended; 4 units over 60 min. This will cover the food consumed over the time interval of that consumption. An additional option is a dual wave bolus/or extended ratio bolus where a percentage of the bolus is given immediately, and the remaining over the extended period. This bolus delivery option is best with food high in fat such as pizza, or cheesecake where the glucose peak absorption is much later.

Manual Alteration in Basal Rates

A temporary basal rate is a reduction or increase of the amount of basal insulin settings during a predefined time, during exercise, fasting, or increased metabolic demand from illness, stress, or medications such as steroids.

Insulin Duration of Action (Becomes the Insulin Onboard)

Insulin duration is the amount of time in hours a dose of bolus of insulin effectively lowers glucose in an individual. This duration of action is programmed into the pump and allows for the pump to determine how much insulin is still "on board" or active. This number is displayed and is subtracted from any insulin calculations needed for correction of a glucose above target or mealtime coverage. This a personalized calculation based on insulin metabolism of the individual. Generally, this number is from 2 to 4 h with up to 5 h. For all automatic insulin delivery, the insulin duration time is fixed at 5 h and cannot be altered. I generally ask the individual how long a bolus of insulin "works" in their body. If they do not know this time action, I generally start at 3 h for that setting and work from there. Let's consider an example, a person has taken a bolus 1 h ago, and they notice an elevated glucose above target. They will put the glucose level into the pump and when the reverse calculation is enabled on the pump the corrective amount of insulin to lower the glucose to target with subtract the amount of insulin currently active. The determined insulin duration allows the pump to display the amount of insulin on board or still active in the persons system. The insulin on board or (IO) then subtracts that amount from any additional calculations for current glycemic level. This prevents stacking insulin or over blousing since there is still insulin working in the system. If a bolus is given manually or without the calculation of the pump, the insulin on board will still display, but there will be no subtraction for the active insulin as the manual essentially goes around this feature. This is why imputing all information such as grams of carb and glucose levels are so essential for successful pumping. I often as the patient are they trusting the pump or are overriding it with the pump between their eyes. For the Tandem with Control IQ algorithm a fixed Insulin duration is 5 h and cannot be adjusted unless suspension of the control IQ feature. The Omnipod 5 and Medtronic pump have programmable insulin duration requirements rather than a pre-fixed level.

Hybrid, Closed-Loop, and Automated Insulin Delivery Systems

The first commercially available hybrid closed-loop system was the Medtronic 670G, FDA approved in September 2016, then the 770G in August 2020.

The Tandem Basal and Control-IQ system was approved by the FDA in 2020 shortly after its tSlim X2 was approved 2019. Other devices continue to be in design and study phases. These include the BetaBionic's iLet system, and Tidepool's Loop Insulet's Omnipod 5 System was released in 2022 and is the most current innovative that is near closed looped.

As of today, the most widely used pump models today in the United States include Medtronic G series, Insulet Omnipod series, and Tandem T-Slim series. Other earlier version of Medtronic, Animas, Tandem, Roche, and recently the Omnipod original series, have virtually been phased out due to support by manufacturer and lack of supply availability. Worldwide there are additional insulin delivery device manufacturers and options but will not be discussed in this publication.

Medtronic 770G and Beyond

As we discussed earlier one of the first systems to integrate CGM and insulin delivery was the Medtronic insulin pump series. Currently, the 770G version is paired with the 10 day Guarding 3 Medtronic continuous glucose sensor. The sensor still requires calibration two times per day, but future CGM versions will most likely eliminate the need for fingerstick. This integrated system prevents, hypoglycemia in 2019, Medtronic started the clinical trials on the MiniMed 780G system, which has enhanced features such as automatic correction boluses, Bluetooth connectivity, and postproduction software updates. This version aims to allow users to achieve a TIR > 80% and a customizable BG target level down to 100 mg/dl. When newer version of the Medtronic pump systems become available, the new software cannot be updated on the current IDD rather the new model pump will need to be purchased [6].

The following information was taken directly from the user manual for the Medtronic MiniMed 770G System on how their glucose algorithm functions.

The starter package consists of the following devices: MiniMed 770G Insulin Pump, the Guardian Link (3) Transmitter, the Guardian Sensor (3), one press inserter, the Accu-Chek Guide Link blood glucose meter, and the Accu-Chek Guide Test Strips. This system is approved for ages 2 and above with sensor insertion location approval abdomen and buttocks and over 14 years of age abdomen and arm. Infusion sets are the MiniMed Quick-set, Sure T, Silhouette, Sure-T and Mio. SmartGuard™ Auto Mode is an insulin delivery feature designed to help people on intensive insulin therapy to achieve better control 24 h a day. This is achieved by automatically controlling basal insulin delivery to regulate glucose levels to a target sensor glucose (SG) amount. The standard target SG setting is 120 mg/dl and the target can be set temporarily to 150 mg/dl for exercise and other events. When Auto Mode is active, the SG values it receives from the transmitter are used to automatically calculate the basal insulin dose. This process of automatic delivery of insulin is called Auto Basal. Auto Mode depends on reliable, accurate sensor measurements and your accurate entry of carbs to deliver insulin for meals. Therefore, the basic management of the therapy requires the following activities: SmartGuard ™ Auto Mode 221 ▪ SmartGuard ™ Auto Mode • Periodic blood glucose (BG) readings using a BG meter to calibrate the sensor. The minimum calibration is every 12 h. For better sensor performance, it is recommended that you calibrate your sensor three or four times each day. You may also receive periodic requests from your pump for BG readings without the need for calibration. • Use of the Auto Mode Bolus feature to deliver boluses to cover meals, and when your pump recommends a bolus [7].

The Medtronic IDD has a maximum fill of 300 unit insulin and is generally changed every 2–3 days. MiniMed™ Mio™ advance infusion set has been approved for extended wear up to 7 days. It has been designed with a new tubing system that can improve the stability of insulin, tubing flow, and limit the immune response at the insertion site. It has an improved adhesive patch, but if users are on more than 300 units in that 7-day period there will need to change the reservoir midway through the site session.

Ominipod 5system Powered by Horizon™

In late 2022, the long awaited Omnipod 5 pump integrated with Dexcom G6 CGM sensor was approved. The Omnipod 5 powered by Horizon™ is termed an AID (Automated Insulin Delivery System) considered the most advanced artificial pancreas available. The Omnipod 5 Horizon™ system is a tubeless patch insulin delivery device that is attached to the skin and infuses insulin through a small plastic flexible canula inserted just under the skin. The pod holds up to 220 units of U100 insulin is attached to the skin using an adhesive and will provide up to 3 days of wear. It delivers insulin for both basal and bolus needs that are programmed into the personal diabetes manager or PDM by the health care provider, such as basal rate, insulin to carb ration, correction factor, and duration of insulin. In addition, the Dexcom G6 CGM displays the glucose value in the PDM and integrates this glucose data into the closed-loop control algorithm build into the Omni pod 5. This closed-loop system will auto correct for additional insulin needed or suspend insulin delivery to prevent hypoglycemia using a predictive glucose algorithm that analyzes the CGM information [8]. Further, after 72 h of initial wear and throughout continuous wear, the Omnipod 5 Horizon™ algorithm is analyzing the glucose and insulin data in the auto mode to create "new pump instructions" based on the trend data. At the tie of writing of this chapter, the Android phone application is available to replace the PDM and has identical functionality and form. The IOS iPhone application is pending release approval from the FDA.

The following information was taken directly from the Omnipod 5 web user information.

SmartAdjust™ technology, Omnipod 5 and the Dexcom G6 Continuous Glucose Monitor are in constant communication, enabling automatic insulin adjustments, every 5 min. The Omnipod 5 Pod is enhanced with a control algorithm called SmartAdjust ™ technology. Every 5 min, SmartAdjust ™ technology receives CGM data and it takes this information and predicts where glucose will be 60 min into the future. It then increases, decreases, or pauses automated insulin using the user's customized Target Glucose settings. The SmartAdjust™

Technology is able to respond to high glucose levels by increasing insulin every 5 min to bring glucose down towards the Target Glucose. Omnipod 5 delivers a micro bolus of insulin every 5 min to reduce blood glucose using the user's customized Target Glucose of 110–150 mg/dl. Automated insulin delivery in the first Pod is initiated based on user-selected basal rate profiles and then adapts over time by tracking insulin delivered by the system. With each new Pod activation, the system adapts insulin delivery based on physiological needs and total daily insulin (TDI) delivered. After 2-3 Pod changes, adaptation generally stabilizes, and automated insulin delivery is based on this adaptation [9].

Currently, the Dexcom G6 in the only CGM system that integrates with the

Omnipod 5. The Dexcom G7 recently released, and the Freestyle Libre 3 are expected to interface in the future.

t:slim X2 Basal and Control IQ Systems by Tandem

The Tandem insulin pump has two control versions that are currently being utilized. The first is the Basal IQ system, where the Dexcom CGM is paired with the IDD and will adjust, or suspended insulin based on the value of the CGM. This model is intended to minimize the risk of hypoglycemia through a glucose predictive algorithm (Fig. 4.2).

The following information was taken directly from the user manual for the Tandem Basal IQ instruction manual on how the algorithm functions.

Basal-IQ technology uses a simple linear regression algorithm that uses Dexcom G6 CGM values to predict glucose levels 30 min ahead based on 3 of the last 4 consecutive CGM readings. If the glucose level is predicted to be <80 mg/dl, or if a CGM reading falls below 70 mg/dl, insulin delivery is suspended. Insulin delivery resumes as soon as sensor glucose values begin to rise. Insulin may be suspended for a minimum of 5 min and a maximum of 2 h within a 2.5-h rolling window.

Shortly after launch of Basal IQ, Tandem made available the software upgrade for Control IQ to current users of the Basal IQ system, with production of its newer

Above 180mg/dl	Correction bolus delivered if glucose predicted to be above 180mg/dl	Delivers
Above 160mg/dl	Increased basal insulin rate if glucose to be above 160mg/dl	B Increases
Between 112.5 and 160 mg/dl	Maintains current profile settings	B Maintains
Less than 112.5 mg/dl	Decreases basal insulin rate if glucose predicted to be below 112.5 mg/dl	B Decreases
Less than 70 mg/dl	Suspension of basal insulin if sensor predicts glucose to be less than 70mg/dl	0 Stops

Fig. 4.2 Tandem control IQ screen icons. Figure Created Dr. Eden Miller DO

of the line pumps running the X2 Control IQ software. In late 2022, yet another updated Tandem control algorithm software upgrade was offered free of charge for those whose pump is currently under warranty, as well as a phone-based app for pump remote control [10].

The following information was taken directly from the user manual for the Tandem Control IQ instruction manual on how the algorithm functions.

Control-IQ technology smoothly decreases or discontinues basal delivery based on falling CGM values to help prevent hypoglycemia. Control-IQ technology helps increase time in range using Dexcom G6 continuous glucose monitoring (CGM)[†] [†] values to predict glucose levels 30 min ahead and adjust insulin delivery, accordingly, including delivery of automatic correction boluses as needed. Every hour it boluses for correction and then run the basal percentage of the total. Control-IQ technology gradually increases basal insulin with increasing CGM values and administers 60% correction boluses once an hour as needed to help prevent hyperglycemia. For Sleep and Exercise Activity Settings Control-IQ technology includes optional settings for Sleep and Exercise Activities that adjust treatment ranges to better match physiologic needs when active or sleeping* [11].

The Tandem t:slim X2 Control IQ system can hold up to 300 units of U100 insulin in the T connect cartridge and currently pairs with the Dexcom CGM series. It is anticipated that the Free Style Libre 3 CGM system and the Dexcom G7 will be able to integrate in the future.

The following are the available infusion set for the tslim X2 pump:

AutoSoft 90 a flexible, 90-degree cannula and automatic inserter.
AutoSoft XC a 90-degree cannula and large grip.

AutoSoft 30 a flexible, 30-degree cannula and automatic inserter.
VariSoft a customizable insertion angle and two choices in cannula length.
TruSteel a 90-degree steel needle and extra adhesive [12].

Do-It-Yourself (DIY) and Super Loopers

The concept of DIY pumping arose out of a group of parents who had heard about the night sentry alert system in development that notified sleeping parents of their child's glucose levels. These parents, not wanting to wait for FDA approval, took it upon themselves to independently develop and engineer the technology or create work around to speed up the availability of new innovations. They named themselves *# we cannot wait*. [These delays inspired parents and computer programmers to create multiple "hacks" for interoperability of several CGM and pump systems prior to FDA clearance. This grass roots movement often used a bridging device to a cell phone application that was open source to remove barriers for initiation. The bridging device would have a price for purchase, but the phone app and information for looping was free. The DIY systems are more customizable but can be time consuming to create. DIY looping uses the CGM, IDD, and these pass-through systems to allow for insulin delivery that is programmable to the user's specifications. There are several resources including *Loopdocs.org* and *CGM in the cloud* Facebook group, where information and guidance for looping can be obtained. More recently, Tidepool loop is the first FDA cleared fully interoperable insulin dosing application [12, 13]. Though some have expressed concern for safety of these systems due to lack of FDA oversite, one must at least pause and acknowledge the passion behind such an undertaking.

Bionic Pancreas (BP)

The "bionic pancreas" is a version of closed-loop system consisting of two simultaneous infusion pumps (one for insulin and the other glucagon). It is considered a dual hormone pump. Its connectivity with a CGM is via a smartphone app that interfaces with the pump algorithm for glycemic control. The first bionic pancreas, "iLet" (Beta Bionics) , is exclusively for T1D persons, was invented by Dr. Edward Damiano in 2015. I spoke with Dr. Damiano personally regarding his invention and was astounded with its capability for a wide range of a1c levels at initiation [14]. The most amazing features of the iLet Bionic pancreas surrounds the onboarding process. Generally, prior to pump initiation, several settings need to be determined, such as total daily dose, hourly basal rates, insulin to carbohydrate ration, correction factor, and insulin duration. iLet's onboarding consists of entering the patient's weight, that is it! Then the user during bolus mealtime periods indicates which meal of the day this is and if that is an average, smaller or larger meal. The iLet takes care of everything else. Reviewing these features literally made my jaw drop. Another, noteworthy thing to mention is iLet's clinical outcome trial data. Beta Bionics' trials demonstrate that all users were able to obtain and A1c of around 7% irrespective of their starting a1c. In other words, iLet's clinical trial included any initial a1c with no upper limit for inclusion in the study. Many other pump clinical trials show a starting a1c level of 7.5–8.3% and at trial completion the a1c improvement was about .5–1% on average. For the iLet users, some individuals had A1c improvement of over 3% and 4%. This bionic pancreas consists of an automated dosing assessments of insulin and glucagon levels are made every 5 min based on the appraised CGM data. These data are transmitted to pumps to regulate insulin or glucagon delivery. Additionally, studies indicated positive psychosocial impacts associated with the use of the bionic pancreas. Another study noted that the insulin-only mode of the iLet (where no glucagon was utilized) there was a significantly increased TIR in adults with type 1 diabetes to 70.1% compared with 61.5% in usual care therapy. Ekhlaspour et al., using a population of T1D patients in the home-use setting, reported that the insulin-only version of the bionic pancreas delivered similar safety and performance outcomes to the other "insulin-only" pumps [15]. The iLet bionic pancreas was granted the "breakthrough device designation" by the FDA in 2019 and will be available in mid-year 2023.

Life Circumstances Such as Exercise, Sleep, and Illness

Exercise or Activity Function

Most insulin delivery devices have the settings options to indicate the person is going to engage in activity such as sleeping or exercising and their needs for insulin will decrease, or they are at an increased risk of hypoglycemia. All CGM integrated pumps have exercise or activity modes that can be activated for the exercise time interval. Additional scenarios where the activity mode can be utilized are time of illness, decreased food intake, or surgical procedures where fasting is required. Using the activity mode can allow for reduction in insulin while remaining in a CGM auto control that prevents hypoglycemia.

Sleep Mode

The Medtronic and Tandem Pumps have a sleep mode feature, that can be activated or scheduled nightly, to avoid nocturnal hypoglycemia. The Omnipod 5 does not have a sleep mode rather its internal algorithm is sufficient to minimize hypoglycemia at during sleep. This feature provides for adjustments in the basal rate, modification of the corrective glucose algorithm which provides less risk of nocturnal hypoglycemia.

Periods of Illness

Sickness can have varying effects on persons with diabetes. Some require additional insulin while others need reduction. While many of the partial or full AID systems have corrective algorithms on board to address hyper- and hypoglycemia, additional insulin navigation may be necessary. As mentioned above for those individuals who tend to have hypoglycemia, using the activity mode minimize this risk. On the flip side, those who experience hyperglycemia, the automated algorithm can generally address the increased insulin needs due to illness. However, it has a threshold for corrective insulin administration, and when the increased insulin needs fall outside these maximum settings, the pump will exit out of automated mode into manual mode where the CGM does not facilitate automated insulin adjustments. This may seem like an undesirable pump design limitation since switching from auto mode to manual mode disables CGM's ability to suspend or increase insulin. This feature is indented to put corrective limits on the pump and require a level of engagement of the person utilizing the pump by not relying on it to be automated in all scenarios. In summary create a sick plan for those using IDD and discuss what the pump can do and what they will be required to do in those conditions.

Essential for Success with IDD/CGM Systems

Downloading and reviewing the ambulatory glucose profile (AGP) and pump report from the online pump manufacturers site. Share and review with this information during the clinical appointment, asking then person what they see in their report or have noticed while using the systems over the past few weeks. Impact hypoglycemia patterns first, then variability, then adjust mealtimes that have the highest peak. Areas of hypoglycemia following times of hyperglycemia can be signs of over correction. When glucoses rise during the day in the unfed state consider increasing that basal segment. Above all, make sure to listen to the person, their concerns, and goals for treatment. After all it's their condition, and we are trying to turn them into experts on their own disease, while addressing the personal barriers to living the best life-taking diabetes along for the ride.

Looking Forward to the Future

As we look to the future of automatic insulin delivery devices paired with continuous glucose monitoring, a few advances are needed to fully replace the dysfunctional pancreas with an external closed-loop system. One of the remaining barriers in insulin delivery devices is the onset of insulin action in the body. These pharmacodynamic and kinetic properties of insulin absorption directly impact the ability to provide physiologic control of insulin/glucose management, either injection or IDD. Rapid-acting analog insulin such as Lispro, Asparts, and Admelog, are preferred in IDD. There are two currently available ultrarapid Lyumjev, and Fiasp have some improved the bioavailability onset of action in the body. These more recent insulin formulations have added components to speed up the absorption and action of the insulin, thus making it more physiologic. To fully acheive the goal of a "fully automated external pancreas," additional inroads to even faster onset insulin need to be developed. Once this is accomplished there will be less of a lag in insulin onset which will minimize glycemic excursion, glucose variability, and improve hypoglycemic rates with more effective insulin suspension [16].

Further advancement in continuous glucose monitoring is ideal; improvement in accuracy, minimal connectivity disruptions, extended on body wear time, and full integration with the available models. Fortunately, as CGM technology advances, all system manufacturers are benefiting. As it is said, high tide raises all boats, and these advances have been the foundation for closed-loop insulin delivery devices. One such advancement is ketone sensors paired or integrated within a continuous glucose monitor. Imagine the ability to detect plasma acetone to prevent the occurrence of diabetic ketoacidosis.

The next necessary advancements are compatibility with other technology innovations such as wearables that track fitness to prevent hypoglycemia, or applications with artificial intelligence with the ability to calculate meal carbohydrates from merely a camera scan of the food. It is exciting to look ahead at the possibility of using technology and artificial intelligence to help restore life back to persons with diabetes.

References

1. Kesavadev J, Saboo B, Krishna MB, Krishnan G. Evolution of insulin delivery devices: from syringes, pens, and pumps to DIY artificial pancreas. Diabetes Ther. 2020;11(6):1251–69.
2. Alsaleh FM, Smith FJ, Keady S, Taylor KM. Insulin pumps: from inception to the present and toward the future. J Clin Pharmacy Ther. 2010;35(2):127–38. https://doi.org/10.1111/j.1365-2710.2009.01048.x.
3. The golden age of the insulin pump by James Hirsch. https://diatribe.org/golden-age-of-the-insulin-pump.
4. Kesavadev J, Saboo B, Krishna MB, Krishnan G. Graphic history of insulin delivery devices. Diabetes Ther. 11(6):1251–69. https://doi.org/10.1007/s13300-020-00831-z.

5. Hiel M, et al. Automated insulin delivery: easy enough to use in primary care. Diabetes Ther. 2020;11(6):1251–69. https://doi.org/10.1007/s13300-020-00831-z.
6. https://www.medtronic.com/us-en/healthcare-professionals/therapies-procedures/diabetes/education/diabetes-digest/extended-infusion-set-and-reservoir.html.
7. https://www.medtronicdiabetes.com/sites/default/files/library/download-library/user-guides/MiniMed_770G_System_User_Guide.pdf.
8. https://www.omnipod.com/current-podders/resources/omnipod5/faqs/smartadjust-technology.
9. Cobry EC, Berget C, Messer LH, Forlenza GP. Review of the Omnipod 5 automated glucose control system powered by Horizon™ for the treatment of type 1 diabetes. Ther Deliv. 2020;11(8):507–19.
10. https://www.tandemdiabetes.com/docs/default-source/product-documents/t-slim-x2-insulin-pump/aw-1005628_d_user-guide-tslim-x2-control-iq-7-4-mgdl-artwork_web.pdf?sfvrsn=18a507d7_217.
11. https://support.tandemdiabetes.com/hc/en-us/articles/1500011451141-How-is-Control-IQ-technology-different-than-Basal-IQ-technology.
12. https://www.tandemdiabetes.com/products/infusion-sets.
13. https://www.tidepool.org/tidepool-loop.
14. Interview with Beta bionic and iLet creator Dr. Edward Damiano 2/8/2023.
15. Ekhlaspour L, Nally LM, El-Khatib FH, Ly TT, Clinton P, Frank E, Tanenbaum ML, Hanes SJ, Selagamsetty RR, Hood K, Damiano ER. Feasibility studies of an insulin-only bionic pancreas in a home-use setting. J Diabetes Sci Technol. 2019;13(6):1001–7. https://doi.org/10.1177/1932296819872225.
16. Templer S. Closed loop insulin delivery systems: past, present, and future direction. Front Endocrinol. 2022;13:919942. https://doi.org/10.3389/fendo.2022.919942/full.

Chapter 5
Continuous Insulin Delivery Systems in the Management of Diabetes Mellitus

Nicholas H. E. Mezitis and Spyros G. E. Mezitis

Introduction

The discovery of insulin in 1922 by Frederick Banting and Charles Best working in Professor John MacCleod's lab in Toronto, Canada, ushered in the new era of diabetes management. Research in the first 50 years since that seminal discovery was centered on sourcing, refining, and commercializing insulin products. Additives permitted modifications in the duration of action of insulin, which was derived from swine or cattle. In 1967, Panayotis Katsoyannis working at Mt. Sinai Hospital in New York achieved the biosynthesis of insulin. This permitted the marketing of a bioidentical "human" insulin product of high purity isolated from microbiota utilizing recombinant technology. Modifications in the structure of the insulin molecule to change its duration of action were soon realized and these "designer" insulin analogues rapidly replaced biosynthetic human insulin in diabetes management.

Research interest then focused on insulin delivery. Technology advances permitted production of ultrafine needles (31 and 32 G) and insulin pens (1985) to replace vials and syringes. Multiple daily injection (MDI) regimens utilizing long-acting

N. H. E. Mezitis (✉)
Ohio University Heritage College of Osteopathic Medicine, Athens, OH, USA

OhioHealth Physician Group Heritage College, Athens, OH, USA

Memorial Health System, Athens, OH, USA

Mezitis Education Research LLC, Athens, OH, USA

S. G. E. Mezitis
Weill Cornell Medical College, New York, NY, USA

New York-Presbyterian Hospital/Weill Cornell Medicine Lenox Hill Hospital/Northwell Health, New York, NY, USA

S. Fishman (ed.), *Advances in Diabetes Technology*, Contemporary Endocrinology, https://doi.org/10.1007/978-3-031-75352-7_5

and short-acting insulin analogues were popularized. Demand also grew for systems that would permit continuous insulin delivery as conceptualized by Arnold Kadish in his 1960s insulin pump.

In 1974, Professor Ernst Pfeiffer in Ulm, Germany working with Miles Laboratories reported on a glucose-controlled (closed-loop) insulin infusion system for diabetes management without dietary restriction. The system became known as the Biostator and its use was restricted to inpatient treatment because of its size and intricacy. Emphasis was placed on miniaturizing pump size and utilizing an open-loop concept. This would permit the patient to decide on bolus insulin delivery to cover for meals or for high blood glucose, while the pump injected insulin continuously at a basal rate (Fig. 5.1).

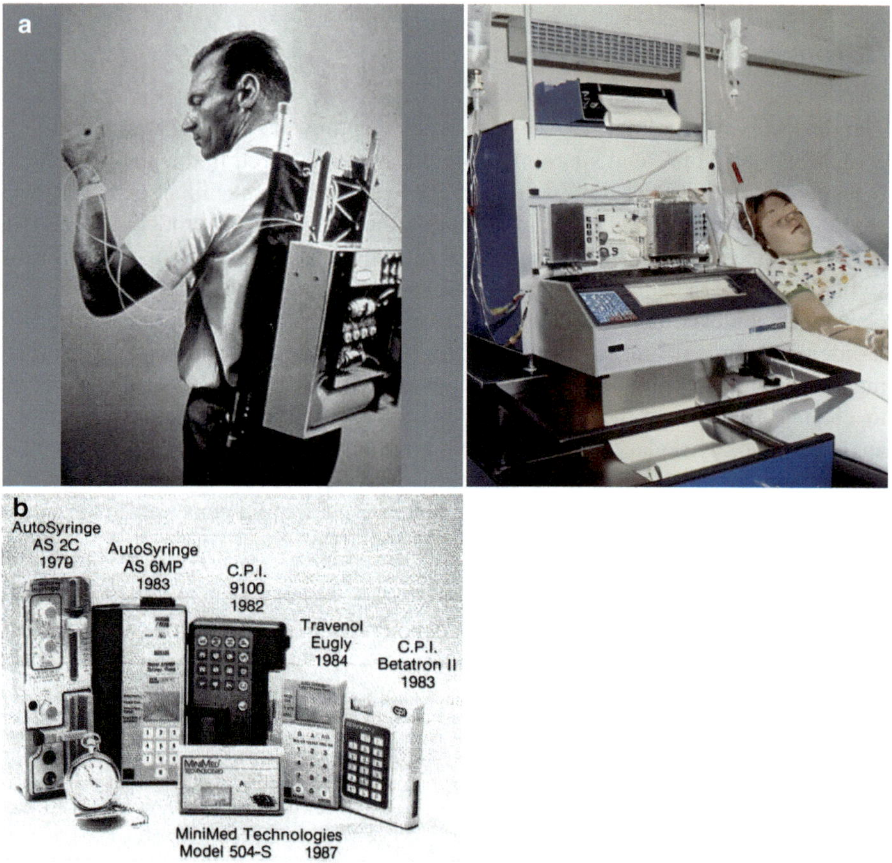

Fig. 5.1 (**a**) Arnold Kadish and his original insulin pump. (**b**) Life Sciences instruments Miles Lab LS 3000RA w/LM86700A Biostator Miles. (**c**) Advances in insulin delivery 1979–1987

Technology achievements in the past 20 years have been exponential and insulin pumps currently in use have a multitude of features. The advent of continuous glucose monitoring in the new millennium has further expanded pump capabilities in optimizing diabetes control.

The conclusion of the Diabetes Control and Complications Trial in the early 1990s confirmed the importance of tight glycemic control, achieved through intensive insulin therapy, in preventing diabetes complications in patients with type 1 diabetes mellitus. This level of control was achieved through a multiple daily insulin injection regimen coupled with frequent capillary blood glucose monitoring. The introduction of continuous subcutaneous insulin infusion (CSII) via pump offered greater comfort and convenience to the patient tasked with maintaining tight diabetes control for a lifetime without sacrificing standards of care. As time proved, glycemic control improved by transitioning patients to automated insulin delivery and episodes of hypoglycemia were less frequent. This led to a surge in pump use in the United States from less than 7000 users in 1990 to over 350,000 users in 2020.

Introduction of continuous glucose monitoring systems (CGMS) and linking their data to the insulin pump has now permitted further optimization of glycemic profiles. As an added benefit, safety features with high and low alarms and predictive algorithms interrupting insulin delivery help prevent emergencies.

Initially limited for use in type 1 diabetes mellitus, insulin pumps are now being increasingly prescribed for patients with type 2 diabetes mellitus as well. The flexibility insulin pumps offer in insulin delivery is of particular value in children and adolescents with their unpredictable eating habits and bursts of physical activity.

Proper selection of candidates for CSII is essential as a level of technical familiarity, motivation, a good support system and hypoglycemia awareness are guarantors of good outcomes.

Current Insulin Pump Technology

Insulin pumps are miniaturized, computerized devices designed to continuously deliver rapid-acting insulin mimicking physiologic insulin release (basal insulin delivery) and to provide a bolus delivery option for mealtime coverage and high glucose correction.

The **basal** infusion of insulin can be set to change its rate with up to 48 basal rates currently possible over the course of a day with some insulin pumps. Alternatively, less frequent changes in basal rate are possible, usually in hourly increments, with some patients electing to have the same basal rate throughout the 24-h period (Table 5.1).

Setting up basal rates for the insulin infusion involves calculating the total daily insulin requirement. One method used for this purpose in adults is to multiply the body weight in kilograms by 0.5. A number of different basal insulin profiles can be

Table 5.1 Commonly used continuous insulin infusion systems

Omnipod: Eros, DASH, and 5 all have 24 basal rates available in each program and up to 12 different programs
Tandem t:slim X2 and Tandem Mobi have 16 rates available in each profile and up to 6 different profiles
Medtronic: 530G, 630G, 670G, 770G, and 780G all have 48 rates available in each basal pattern and up to 8 basal patterns

pre-programmed into the insulin pump to conform to variations in activities of daily living, for example, "sick days," sport, holiday, workday, etc.

Bolus doses of insulin can be delivered with meals based on calculations taking the insulin: carbohydrate ratio (ICR), correction algorithms (insulin sensitivity ratio, ISR), and target blood glucose into account. Built-in calculators may consider insulin remaining from previous boluses and the patient's insulin action time in suggesting an insulin dose for meal coverage. This open-loop system provides the option for the patient to override the suggested bolus dose. Bolus doses may also be given for correction purposes, independently of meals.

Bolus insulin delivery is required to control postprandial blood glucose excursions. Instruction in carbohydrate counting permits the patient to enter an accurate estimate of their meal composition. Information regarding the actual blood glucose level at the time of the meal allows the pump to add a correction dose to the dose calculated from the insulin carbohydrate ratio. The glucose result may be entered by the patient based on capillary blood glucose testing. Increasingly, this data is provided by a continuous transdermal glucose monitoring sensor communicating with the pump.

The formula to calculate the initial **insulin to carbohydrate ratio** equals 450 divided by the total daily insulin dose. The **insulin sensitivity factor** on which the correction dose is calculated is obtained initially by dividing 1700 by the total daily insulin requirement.

The insulin carbohydrate ratio and the insulin sensitivity ratio may vary at times during the day. For simplicity, when initiating continuous subcutaneous insulin delivery (CSII) therapy a single ICR and ISR are utilized together with a single basal rate.

Basal rates and bolus settings may be later modified by defining time limits based on the glucose profile data.

The risk from over frequent corrections (insulin stacking) and hypoglycemia is minimized by the preset memory feature which calculates the residual bolus insulin activity from the last insulin dose (an estimation of how much insulin is still active in the body).

There are three types of insulin pumps currently on the market.

1. The patch insulin pump attaches directly to the surface of the skin and has controls on the pump itself (V-Go) or on a remote control (OmniPod). There is no tubing with these pumps, and they are safe for water immersion. The V-Go and the OmniPod Go and the OmniPod are the only commercially available patch

pumps in the United States, with the former two having only limited features which accounts for their FDA classification as an "insulin delivery device" rather than as a bona fide "insulin pump." Of note, the CeQur Simplicity was recently approved as an insulin patch device designed to deliver bolus insulin doses only (2 units/click) for meals or correction purposes.

2. The tethered insulin pumps have flexible tubing between the pump and the cannula which is inserted into the skin. The pump features controls and it can be tucked into pockets or carried in special pouches which can be worn under or outside of clothing. Commercially available tethered insulin pumps are the Medtronic 530G, 630G, 670G, 770G, 780G, and the Tandem t:slim and Tandem Mobi.
3. The implanted insulin pump is placed in the peritoneal cavity and requires access to special centers for insulin refill. Their use is limited (Figs. 5.2, 5.3, 5.4 and 5.5).

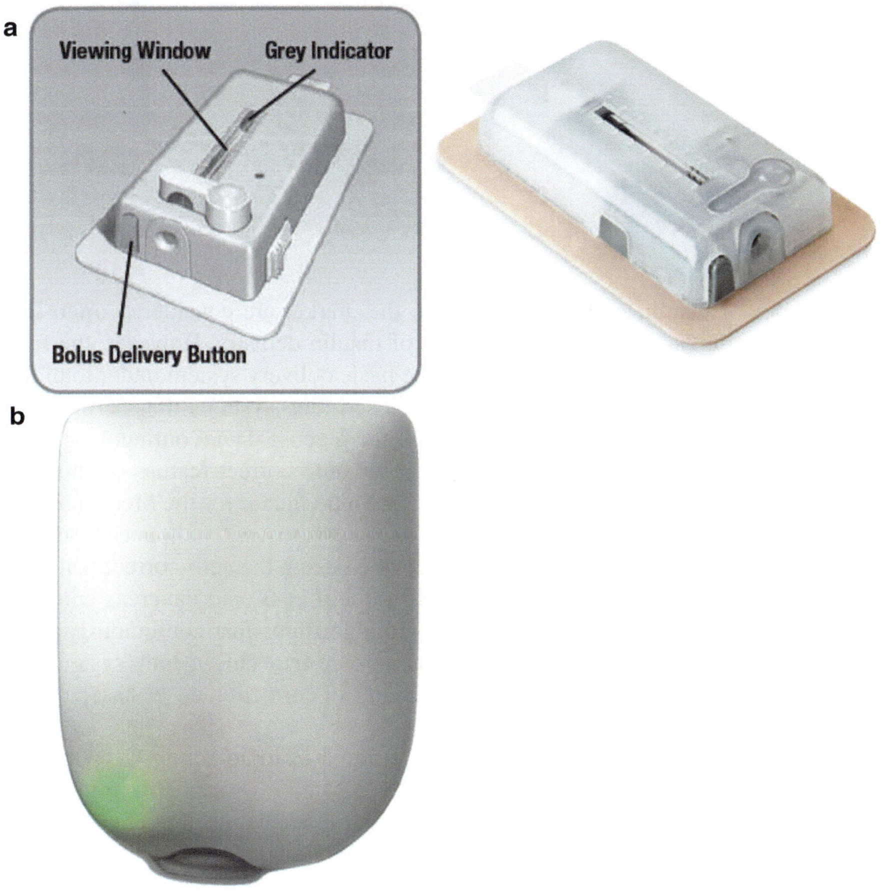

Fig. 5.2 (**a**) The V-Go system. (**b**) The Omnipod GO system

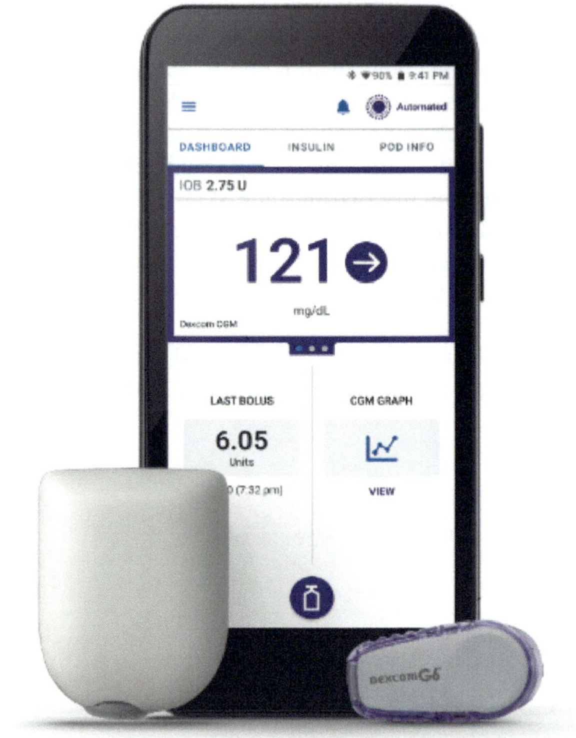

Fig. 5.3 The Omnipod G5 system (integrates with Dexcom G6 and Dexcom G7)

All types of insulin pumps currently on the market are considered **open-loop** devices since the patient maintains control of insulin delivery. However, the functional aspects of insulin pumps vary from the basic delivery system under total user control to the increasingly popular hybrid closed-loop systems that permit automatic adjustment in basal rate based on real-time glucose data (continuous glucose monitoring system) and preset parameters. This auto-correct feature is known as Smart Adjust for the Omnipod 5, AutoMode or Smart Guard for the Medtronic, and Control IQ or Smart IQ for the Tandem-T slim. Users must still announce meals and exercise and estimate carbohydrate amounts when using the auto-correct feature.

Next-generation technology represented by the iLet Bionic Pancreas automatically deliver insulin based on sensor data and algorithms that continuously adjust insulin dose based on user's needs. These devices are **true closed-loop** systems that do not require carbohydrate counting or estimates of correction doses based on glucose monitoring by the patient.

The V-GO patch pump contains a preset amount of rapid-acting U-100 insulin (20, 30, or 40 units) for continuous delivery over 24 h, as well as 36 extra units for optional bolus delivery. It represents a convenient mode of insulin delivery for the patient with type 2 diabetes mellitus and is replaced daily.

The OmniPod GO, recently approved, features a tubeless, waterproof pod that provides a fixed rate of basal insulin delivery in one of seven pre-programmed basal

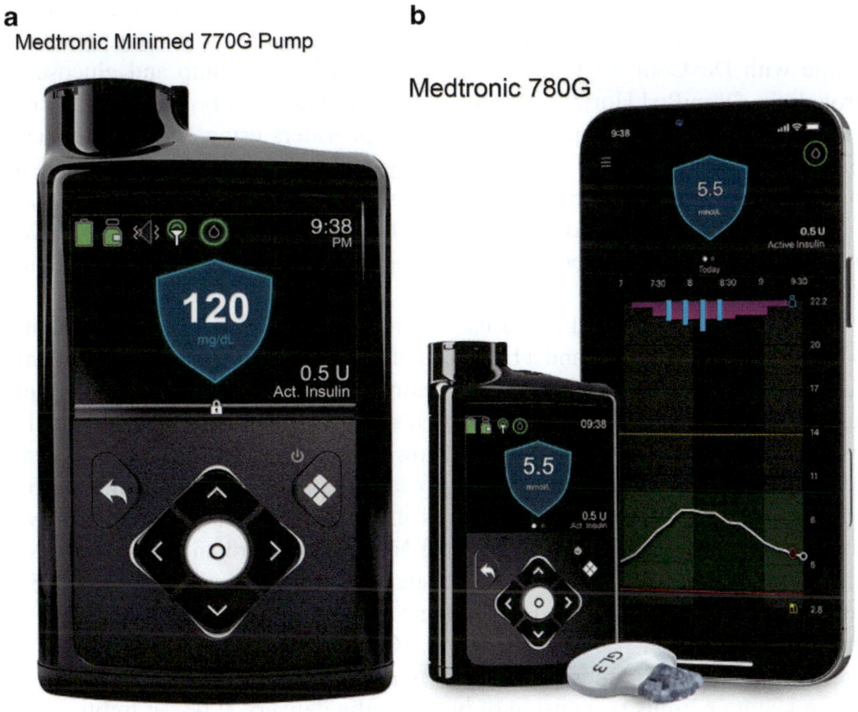

Fig. 5.4 (a) Medtronic Minimed 770G Insulin pump. (b) Medtronic Minimed 780G Insulin pump

Fig. 5.5 Tandem Diabetes Care: T-slim X2 Control-IQ Pump

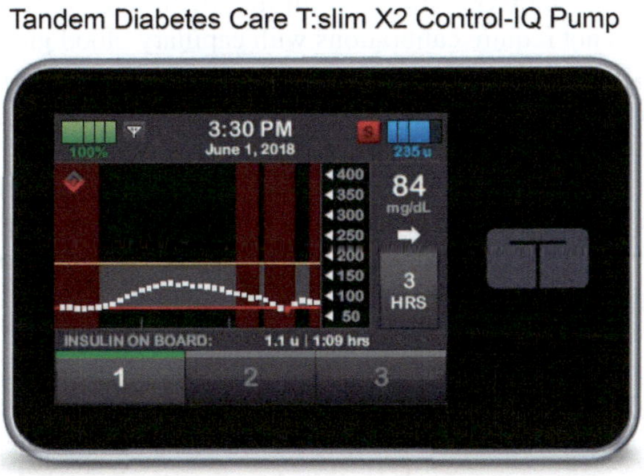

rates ranging from 10 to 40 units per day. It operates without the need for a handheld device to control the pod.

The OmniPod DASH and OmniPod 5 patch pump have a reservoir for 200 units of U-100 rapid-acting insulin and may remain in situ for up to 72 h. They are remotely monitored and adjusted by a Controller, formerly known as a Personal

Diabetes Management device, which has a bolus calculator. An integrated food library database is available in some models. The OmniPod 5 is smartphone compatible with DexCom 6 CGMS connectivity, integrating pump and glucose data through the OmniPod Horizon algorithm to adjust basal and bolus insulin delivery. Reports can be communicated to health care providers using Android phones for commentary. Software can also be remotely updated through secure connection. Patients with insulin requirements in excess of 200 U/day have used U-200 and U-500 rapid-acting insulin off-label in the OmniPod reservoir. The pump is waterproof for up to 25 ft. deep for 60 min avoiding the need to disconnect for swimming or bathing.

The Medtronic Minimed 530G uses tubing. It has a reservoir for 300 units of U-100 rapid-acting insulin and a bolus calculator. An optional glucometer (Contour Next) can transmit data to the pump. Continuous glucose monitoring is an option through the Medtronic Enlite CGM which communicates with the pump and can suspend basal insulin delivery if a preset low glucose threshold triggers the system.

An improvement in the tethered pump series is the Medtronic Minimed 670G which has a similar reservoir capacity as its predecessor but can act as a hybrid closed-loop system when it links with the Medtronic Guardian Sensor 3 CGM. In this mode, automated adjustments may be made to the basal insulin rate every 5 min based on CGM readings to maintain a target blood glucose at the provider's discretion, usually between 100 and 150 mg/dL. Calibration of the glucose sensor with capillary blood glucose measurements is required at least fourt times daily. A predictive feature permits suspension of basal insulin delivery at preset limits to avoid hypoglycemia. Restart on recovery in profile is automatic with a 2-h lag or manual by the user. The bolus calculator is a feature here as well. The Guardian Sensor 4 is an updated CGM for use with the Medtronic 780G recently approved. The 780G does not require calibrations with capillary blood glucose testing.

The main differentiating features for this new pump are the auto-correct feature that delivers small auto boluses for blood glucose above threshold activated independently and the flexibility in glucose targets which can be 100, 110, or 120 mg/dL.

Medtronic pumps of the 500 and 600 series are designated as "splash-proof" in their manuals. The Medtronic 770G is described as "waterproof." Water immersion to 12 ft. for up to 24 h at a time is possible, but not recommended by the manufacturer.

Medtronic has now introduced an extended-wear infusion set and reservoir holding up to 300 units of rapid-acting insulin designed for twice the wear time. New materials used for the reservoir reduce the risk of line occlusion maintaining insulin stability.

The Tandem t:slim X2 is a tethered pump with software that can be uploaded remotely from a computer. The Tandem t:slim X2 has a reservoir for 300 U of U-100 rapid-acting insulin. It has a bolus calculator. Immersion in up to 3 ft. of water for up to 30 min is permitted.

The Tandem t:slim X2 has touch screen capability and can be used independently or with a Dexcom CGM. Using the Dexcom 6 CGM permits trend monitoring on the pump screen and the setting of high and low alerts as well as predictive basal insulin delivery suspension at preset limits and automatic restart on recovery. Tandem t:slim X2 has two features/upgrades: Basal IQ and Control IQ. Basal IQ technology will decrease the basal rate if the BG is predicted to be below 112.5 mg/dL and would automatically stop all insulin delivery if BG was predicted to go below 70 mg/dL. Control IQ has the automatic basal adjustment for low (like the Basal IQ) but will also increase basal rate if BG is predicted to be above 160 mg/dL and can also deliver a small bolus if BG is predicted to be greater than 180 mg/dL. A bolus can be repeated every hour if needed.

Dexcom 6 CGM is currently approved for use with the OmniPod 5, Tandem t:slim X2, Tandem Mobi, and iLet Beta Bionic insulin pumps. Data may be shared in real time with up to five caregivers using Apple or Android devices. Glucose alerts for followers can be customized to permit timely intervention.

Dexcom 7 CGM pairs with FreeStyle Libre 2, Tandem t:slim X2, and iLet Beta Bionic (Figs. 5.6, 5.7, 5.8, 5.9, 5.10 and 5.11; Tables 5.2, 5.3 and 5.4).

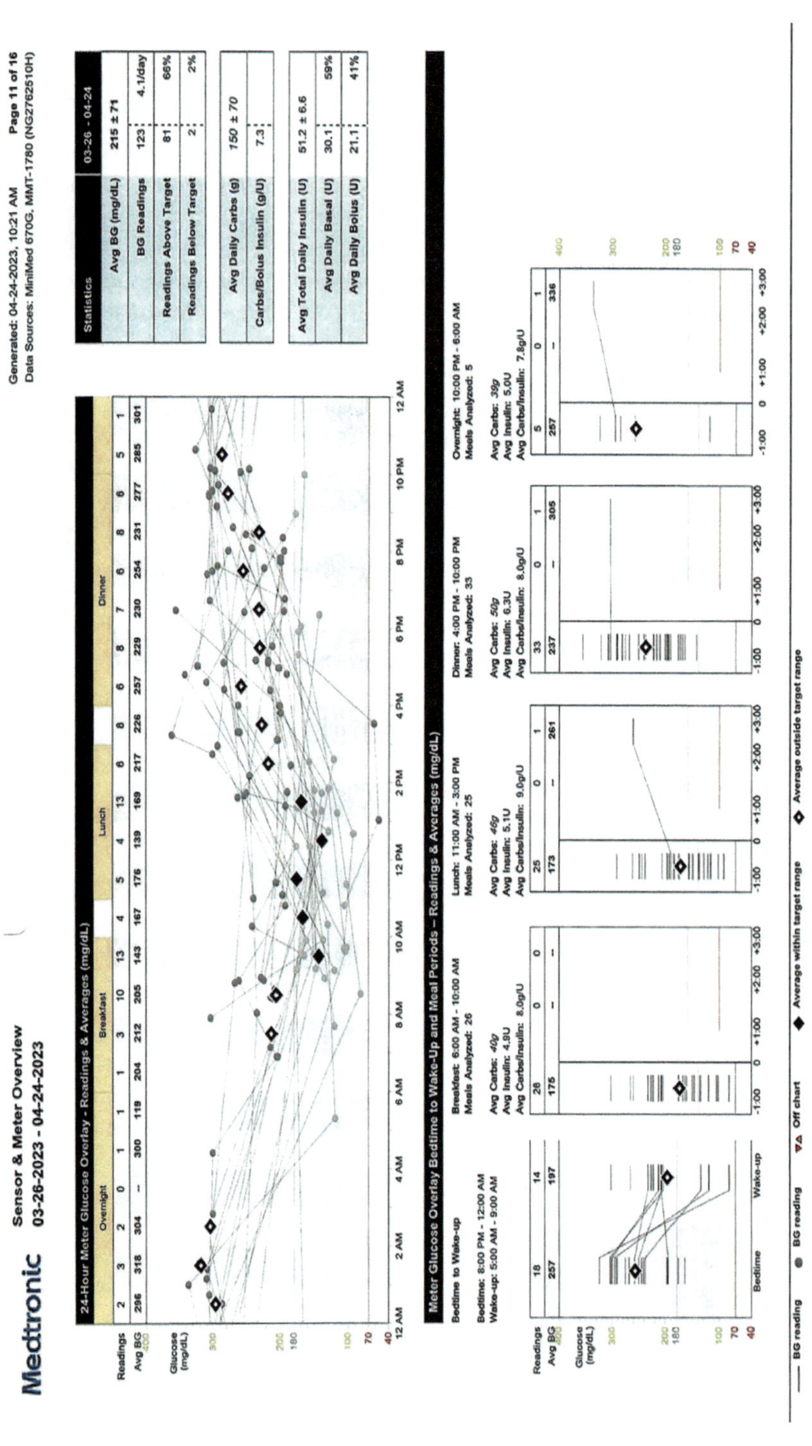

Fig. 5.6 Sampled Medtronic Insulin pump report. Meter/sensor overview display: information on meal number, carbohydrate distribution, readings above and below target, total daily carbohydrate consumption (average), average total daily insulin (basal and bolus)

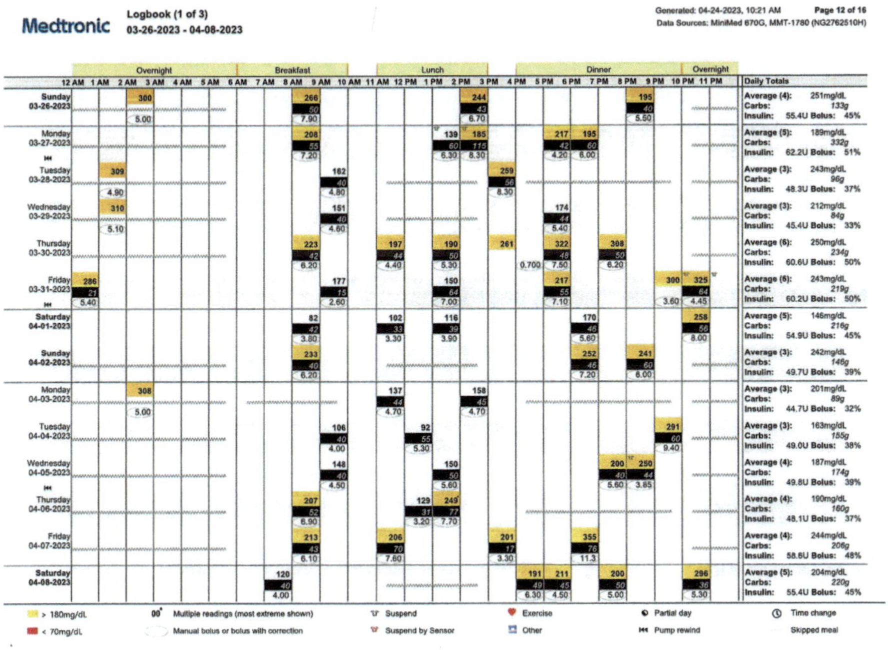

Fig. 5.7 Medtronic Logbook sample. Logbook: Features blood glucose at time of bolus, bolus dose, carbohydrates consumed (individual meal and daily total), insulin (mealtime bolus and daily total)

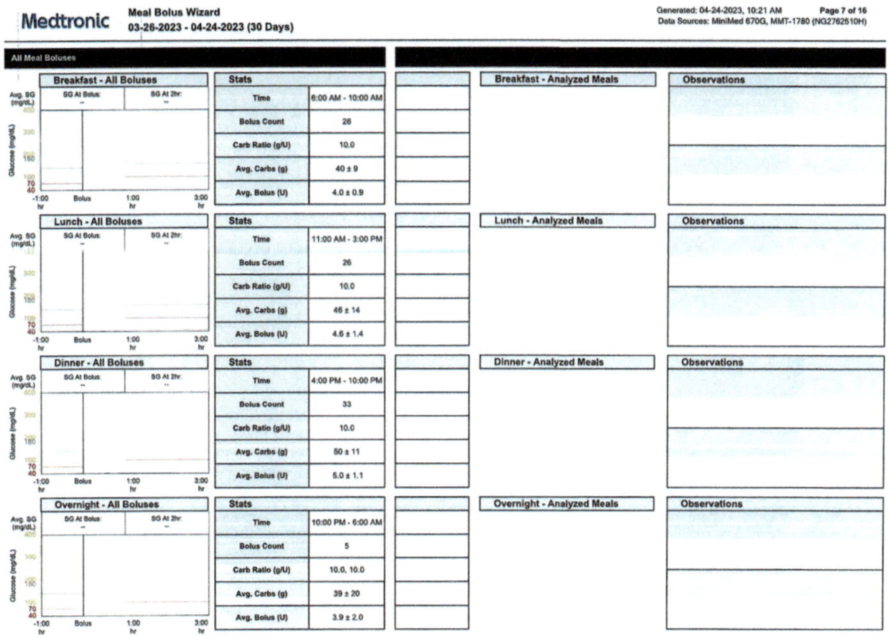

Fig. 5.8 Medtronic meal bolus calculator. Meal bolus calculator: Number of meals, insulin: carbohydrate ratio (ICR), average carbohydrates/mealtime, average bolus delivered (based on ICR)

Medtronic Adherence (1 of 3)
03-26-2023 - 04-08-2023

Generated: 04-24-2023, 10:21 AM Page 8 of 16
Data Sources: MiniMed 670G, MMT-1780 (NG2762510H)

	Glucose Measurements		Bolus Events					Fill Events					
	BG Readings	Sensor Duration (h:mm)	Manual Boluses	Bolus Wizard Events	With Food	With Correction	Overridden	Rewind	Cannula Fills	Cannula Amount (U)	Tubing Fills	Tubing Amount (U)	Suspend Duration (h:mm)
Sunday 03-26-2023	4			4	3	4	1						
Monday 03-27-2023	5			6	6	6	1	1	1	0.6	1	6.0	0:04
Tuesday 03-28-2023	3			3	2	3	1						
Wednesday 03-29-2023	3			3	2	3	1						
Thursday 03-30-2023	6			6	5	6							
Friday 03-31-2023	6			6	5	6	1	1	1	0.6	1	13.7	0:16
Saturday 04-01-2023	5			5	5	3							
Sunday 04-02-2023	3			3	3	3							
Monday 04-03-2023	3			3	2	3	1						
Tuesday 04-04-2023	3			3	3	2							
Wednesday 04-05-2023	4			4	4	4	1	1	1	0.6	1	8.7	0:05
Thursday 04-06-2023	4			4	4	4							
Friday 04-07-2023	4			4	4	4							
Saturday 04-08-2023	5			5	5	4							
Summary	4.1/day	0m	0.0/day	4.2/day	89.8%	93.2%	11.9%	3	3	0.6U /fill	3	9.5U /fill	25m

Partial day   Suspend   Suspend On Low   Suspend Before Low

Fig. 5.9 Medtronic activity calculator. Activity profile: Depicts number of glucose readings accessed, food (carbohydrate) entries, bolus delivered, readings not covered with insulin (overridden), pump refills, pump suspensions

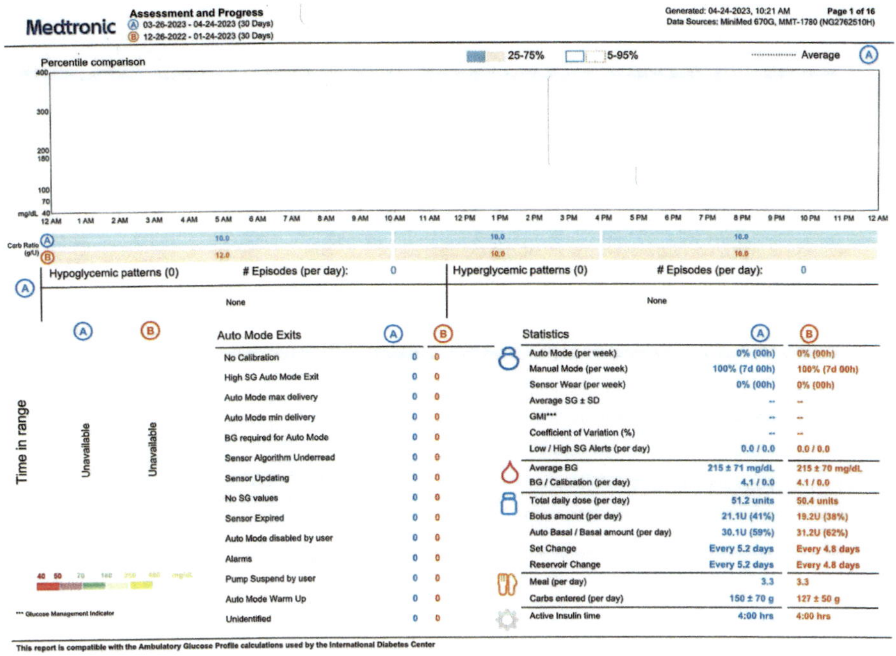

Fig. 5.10 Medtronic activity progress report. Progress report: patterns of insulin delivery, glucose trends above and below target range, average blood glucose results insulin delivery totals, reservoir changes (refills), average number of meals consumed, active insulin time (blocks additional bolus)

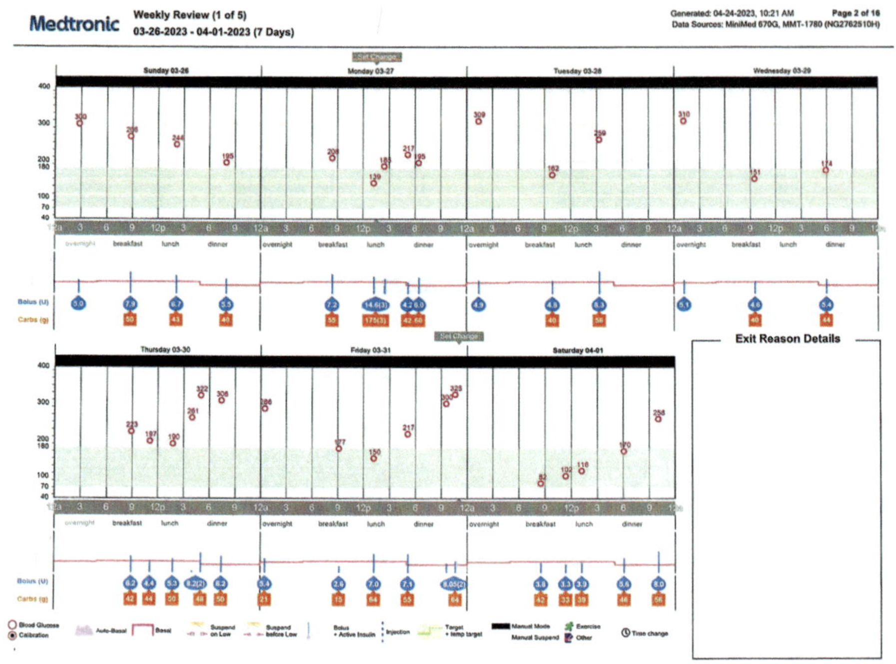

Fig. 5.11 Medtronic weekly overview report. Weekly overview: displays daily glucose trends with results corresponding to times data were accessed, features insulin dose delivered, markings for basal insulin delivery, exercise, pump suspensions, operation in manual or auto-basal mode

Table 5.2 Online resources for adjusting insulin pump settings

How to look up pump setting and adjust basal rate and bolus setting
Tandem: T-slim X2: Personal profiles: https://www.youtube.com/watch?v=wpz8Da0DU_w
Omnipod: Basal rate change: https://www.youtube.com/watch?v=X0GbyZ3u-ac Bolus calculator (carb ratio, correction factor, target BG): https://www.youtube.com/watch?v=o-x4D8AnQNs
Omnipod DASH: Basal rate changes: https://www.youtube.com/watch?v=Gvq7Kv87Dnc Bolus calculator (carb ratio, correction factor, target BG): https://www.youtube.com/watch?v=jkbz-VnDdFE
Omnipod 5: The instruction to "switch" modes starts on time frame 2:01, if you want to skip to this point: https://www.omnipod.com/current-podders/resources/omnipod-5/videos/automated-mode

(continued)

Table 5.2 (continued)

How to look up pump setting and adjust basal rate and bolus setting
Basal rate change: https://www.youtube.com/watch?v=BnF6JlpyVI0 Bolus calculator changes: https://www.omnipod.com/current-podders/resources/omnipod-5/videos/bolus-setting-editing
Medtronic: MiniMed 530G, 630G, 670G, 770G, 780G: All the pumps available on this link—these are written steps: https://www.medtronicdiabetes.com/customer-support/device-settings-and-features/basal-settings/basal-rate

iLet Beta Bionic: www.betabionics.com

Table 5.3 Types of insulin pump algorithms

Types of insulin pump algorithms
1. Open-loop algorithms: These algorithms use pre-programmed settings to deliver insulin based on a person's current blood glucose level and the time of day. They do not take into account the person's recent insulin dose history or individual insulin sensitivity
2. Closed-loop algorithms: Also known as "artificial pancreas" systems, these algorithms use real-time blood glucose monitoring to automatically adjust the amount of insulin being delivered through the pump. They can also take into account the person's recent insulin dose history and insulin sensitivity to more accurately deliver insulin
3. Hybrid closed-loop algorithms: These algorithms are a combination of open-loop and closed-loop systems, allowing the person to make some manual adjustments while still benefiting from automatic insulin delivery
4. Adaptive closed-loop algorithms: These algorithms are initialized only with a user's body weight and blood glucose target range. Meal announcements are entered

Table 5.4 Considerations for successful insulin pump candidates

• Patients on multiple daily insulin injections
• Patients using CGMS and using insulin who wish to improve their glycemic profile
• Patients with technical familiarity utilizing smartphones and computers
• Patients comfortable wearing devices on a 24 h basis
• Patients with a good support system, for example, family members, partners, health care personnel
• Patients willing to perform frequent capillary blood glucose monitoring, as needed
• Patients comfortable with carbohydrate counting and correction dose calculations
• Patients prepared to cooperate with health care personnel in communicating data and following instructions
• Patients willing to attend education sessions for pump use and diabetes management
• Patients with health insurance coverage or financial resources to support costs for insulin delivery technology and glucose monitoring
• Special provisions with appropriate technology/pump features (predictive alarms) for patients with hypoglycemia unawareness

Insulins, Insulin Analogues, and Biosimilars in Insulin Pump Therapy

Early insulins were crudely refined acidic formulations from animal sources with concentrations of <10 units/mL. Continuous improvement in chemical engineering provided us insulins with concentrations 100 U/mL (U-100). More recently bioengineering has developed bioidentical human insulin from microbiota, as well as insulin analogues ("designer insulins") with special features. These products provide us with choices in onset and duration of action, as well as choices in concentration, for example, U-200, U-300, or U-500. Concentration is of particular importance in limiting injection volume in insulin-resistant patients requiring high doses of insulin. Understanding the insulin armamentarium permits bespoke therapy for patients according to their special circumstances.

Short-acting biosynthetic human insulin (Humulin or Novolin) or rapid-acting insulin analogues (lispro, aspart, glulisine) have all been used in insulin pumps.

Insulin analogues are now preferred for use in insulin pumps because of their rapid onset of action. Differences in interruptions in insulin flow due to occlusion in the tubing are a feature that may influence choice [1]. Bode et al. [2] used low flow rates over 5 days in a non-clinical setting to show probabilities for occlusion with lispro (15.7%), aspart (9.2%), and glulisine (40.9%). All occlusions occurred after 48 h of pump use and mostly during bolus infusion. Occlusion alarms were delayed at low infusion rates by as much as 24 h. Zisser et al. [3] demonstrated that in pump shut off the blood glucose level rises by approximately 1 mg/dL/min for the first 30 min of occlusion.

Insulin pharmacokinetics has been influenced by locally warming the infusion site, which accelerates subcutaneous insulin delivery. Raz et al. [4] have reported on a local heating device which significantly decreased *T*(max) and *T* (50% max) and increased insulin AUC and *C* (max) of subcutaneously infused rapid-acting insulin analogues.

Long-acting insulins (glargine, detemir, or degludec) are provided to insulin pump patients for use in emergencies when the insulin pump needs to be removed. These substitute for the insulin pump basal delivery mode, while the rapid-acting insulin analogue is dosed based on the scale (insulin:carb ratio and insulin:sensitivity ratio) programmed into the insulin pump.

Human regular U-500 insulin has been used successfully in "open-loop" insulin pump therapy. Safe use is facilitated by delivery in a specially calibrated pump such as the Omnipod DASH U-500 Insulin management System (Insulet Corporation, Acton, MA, USA) as reported by Grunberger et al. [5].

Insulin Pump Supplies and Costs

Pump sets include the pump device, flexible needles for insertion of the infusion line, infusion lines, and adhesive for securing the infusion line. Some sets include a clip-on belt or pouch for the pump and computer software to connect the device with a personal computer or smartphone.

Expenses for insulin pump therapy include the cost of the pump and the cost of infusion lines, cartridges, reservoirs, syringes, batteries, pods, and insulin. Additionally, one must factor in the cost of glucose monitoring supplies (strips and glucometers or CGMS and sensors).

Medical follow-up involves consultation on a regular basis with specialists and support staff experienced in insulin pump therapy.

Insurance may cover these costs in part, but gaps in coverage may result in significant expense.

Non-profit groups as well as state and federal agencies offer help with prescription cost for qualifying individuals. The Partnership for Prescription Assistance helps patients, and their families locate these programs at no cost.

The American Diabetes Association offers a resource guide for individual pumps, insulin options and infusion sets (https://consumerguide.diabetes.org/collections/pumps).

The Importance of a Back-Up Plan ("Plan B") in Insulin Pump Therapy

Insulin pump therapy offers remarkable flexibility in diabetes management, which when properly supervised can help the patient improve their glycemic profile. The present systems, however, place a burden of responsibility on the patient who must participate in meal decisions and calculate carbohydrate load as well as plan for physical activity in order to inform insulin bolus delivery [6].

Successful candidates for insulin pump therapy have usually mastered meal planning and carbohydrate counting (Gillespie et al. https://doi.org/10.1016/S0002-8223(98)00206-5) and are familiar with multiple daily insulin injection (MDI) regimens using long-acting (basal) and rapid-acting (bolus) insulin analogues. Transition to the insulin pump introduces the convenience of continuous subcutaneous insulin infusion (CSII) using only rapid-acting insulin. Glycemic control improves and the patient is freed of carrying insulin pens, vials, and syringes as they engage in their daily activities. Insulin delivery is discreet and reliable.

Familiarity with multiple daily insulin injection (MDI) management is essential in order to permit seamless transition off the insulin pump, if need arises (Plan B). Patients are instructed to discontinue use of their pump if blood glucose results are increasing unchecked and there are questions about reliable insulin delivery. Making changes to the insulin pump and its attachments while in such a situation may delay

Table 5.5 Insulin correction table

Example: Glucose in target range 80–120 mg/dL take insulin based on ICR. Adjust for glucose above target range (mg/dL)			
	Child	Adolescent/ adult	Adolescent/adult (insulin-resistant)
121–150	+0.5 U	+1 U	+2 U
151–200	+1 U	+2 U	+4 U
201–250	+1.5 U	+3 U	+6 U
251–300	+2 U	+4 U	+8 U
301–350	+2.5 U	+5 U	+10 U
351–400	+3 U	+6 U	+12 U
>400 notify diabetes support team			

insulin delivery and lead to DKA. Once the glycemic profile has improved on MDI, return to the insulin pump may be planned in collaboration with the supervising health care provider team.

In preparation for such eventualities, patients are prescribed a long-acting insulin which is stored for use as needed. The dose will reflect the total 24 h basal insulin requirement in the pump settings. Our preference is to split the amount of long-acting insulin into two equal doses delivered 10–12 h apart. The bolus injection will use the patient's rapid-acting insulin with calculation based on the insulin:carb ratio (ICR) and a correction scale. The correction scale in our practice adjusts based on age (child vs. adolescent/adult) and level of insulin resistance (low or high) (Table 5.5).

The Future of Insulin Pump Therapy

Sensor-augmented pump (SAP) therapy has provided a significant advance in optimizing glycemic profiles. In an SAP system, the insulin pump pairs to the continuous glucose monitoring system (CGM) permitting not only the display of glucose information on the pump screen, but also the modulation of **basal insulin delivery** within predetermined parameters and the suspension of basal insulin delivery for hypoglycemia or hypoglycemia trend.

The next step in this technology is research in perfecting a true "closed loop" pump system which would permit full automation in **bolus insulin delivery** based on users' needs and their body weight. Algorithms to make these calculations rely on accurate blood glucose determinations through sampling of interstitial fluid and entrain to the glycemic profile in response to meals, obviating the need for carbohydrate counting [7].

Subcutaneous insulin delivery remains a limiting feature in insulin pump therapy in contradistinction to the physiologic delivery of endogenous insulin directly to the liver through the portal system. Bathing the tissues in supraphysiologic concentrations of insulin and insulin analogues in order to adequately insulinize the liver may harbor risks [8, 9].

Alternate routes of insulin delivery such as intraperitoneal or intraportal with implantable pumps have been investigated and may be realized in future systems [10, 11, 12].

Dual hormone (glucagon and insulin) delivery devices are also being investigated and may have a role in future management of diabetes mellitus with closed-loop systems [13].

Acknowledgments William Mezitis, Junior at Bronx Science High School, Technical Advisor for Insulin Pump Technology. Lora Shaner, RN. Diabetes Educator. Marietta Memorial Health System. Steve Wang, Information Technology Consultant.

References

1. Klonoff DC, et al. J Diabetes Sci Technol. 2017;11(3):451–4.
2. Bode BW. Endocr Pract. 2011;17(2):271–80.
3. Zisser H. Diabetes Care. 2008;31(2):238–9.
4. Raz I. Clin Ther. 2009;31(5):980–7.
5. Grunberger G, et al. Diabetes Obes Metab. 2020;22(3):434–41.
6. Simon B, et al. Int J Clin Pract. 2008;62(12):1858–63.
7. Bionic Pancreas Research Group. N Engl J Med. 2022;387:1161–72.
8. Regittnig W, Tschaikner M, et al. Diabetes Obes Metab. 2022;24(3):455–64.
9. Soares S, Costa A, Sarmento B. Exp Opin Drug Deliv. 2012;9(12):1539–58.
10. Dassau E, Renard E, et al. Diabetes Obes Metab. 2017;19(12):1698–705.
11. SaudekC,etal.DiabetesEduc.1989;15(1):44–9.https://doi.org/10.1177/014572178901500112.
12. Udelsman R, Chen H, Loman K, Pitt HA, Saudek CD. Surgery. 1997;122(6):10005–1011.
13. Lindkvist EB, et al. Performance of a dual-hormone closed-loop system versus insulin-only closed-loop system in adolescents with type 1 diabetes. A single-blind, randomized, controlled, crossover trial. Front Endocrinol (Lausanne). 2023;14:1073388.

Further Reading

Banting FG, Best CH. The internal secretion of the pancreas. 1922. Indian J Med Res. 2007;125:251–66.

Lewis GF, Brubaker PL. The discovery of insulin revisited: lessons for the modern era. J Clin Invest. 2021;131(1):e142239.

Nathan DM. Long-term complications of diabetes mellitus. N Engl J Med. 1993;328:1676–85.

Nathan DM, for the DCCT/EDIC Research Group. The diabetes control and complications trial/epidemiology of diabetes interventions and complications study at 30 years: overview. Diabetes Care. 2014;37(1):9–16.

Templer S. Closed-loop insulin delivery systems: past, present, and future directions. Front Endocrinol. 2022;13:919942.

DCCT Research Group, Nathan DM, Genuth S, Lachin J, et al. The effect of intensive treatment of diabetes on the development and progression of long-term complications in insulin-dependent diabetes mellitus. N Engl J Med. 1993;329:977–86.

Fry A. Insulin delivery device technology 2012: where are we after 90 years? J Diabetes Sci Technol. 2012;6:947–53.

Bode BW, Sabbah HT, Gross TM, Fredrickson LP, Davidson PC. Diabetes management in the new millennium using insulin pump therapy. Diabetes Metab Res Rev. 2002;18(Suppl 1):S14–20.
Nathan DM, Cleary PA, Backlund JY, et al., DCCT/EDIC Research Group. Intensive diabetes treatment and cardiovascular disease in patients with type 1 diabetes. N Engl J Med. 2005;353:2643–53.
McAdams BH, Rizvi AA. An overview of insulin pumps and glucose sensors for the generalist. J Clin Med. 2016;5:5.
Miller KM, Foster NC, Beck RW, et al., TID Exchange Clinic Network. Current state of type 1 diabetes treatment in the U.S.: updated data from the T1D Exchange Clinic Registry. Diabetes Care. 2015;38:971–8.
Reznik Y, Cohen O. Insulin pump for type 2 diabetes: use and misuse of continuous subcutaneous insulin infusion in type 2 diabetes. Diabetes Care. 2013;36(Suppl 2):S219–25.
Bode BW. Insulin pump use in type 2 diabetes. Diabetes Technol Ther. 2010;12(Suppl. 1):S17–21.
Alsaleh FM, Smith FJ, Taylor KM. Experiences of children/young people and their parents, using insulin pump therapy for the management of type 1 diabetes: qualitative review. J Clin Pharm Ther. 2012;37:140–7.
Weissberg-Benchell J, Antisdel-Lomaglio J, Seshadri R. Insulin pump therapy: a meta-analysis. Diabetes Care. 2003;26:1079–87.
Burckhardt MA, Smith GJ, Cooper MN, Jones TW, Davis EA. Real-world outcomes of insulin pump compared to injection therapy in a population-based sample of children with type 1 diabetes. Pediatr Diabetes. 2018;19:1459–66.
Mameli C, Scaramuzza AE, Ho J, Cardona-Hernandez R, Suarez-Ortega L, Zuccotti GV. A 7-year follow-up retrospective, international, multicenter study of insulin pump therapy in children and adolescents with type 1 diabetes. Acta Diabetol. 2014;51:205–10.
Brorsson AL, Viklund G, Ortqvist E, Lindholm Olinder A. Does treatment with an insulin pump improve glycaemic control in children and adolescents with type 1 diabetes? A retrospective case-control study. Pediatr Diabetes. 2015;16:546–53.
Litton J, Rice A, Friedman N, Oden J, Lee MM, Freemark M. Insulin pump therapy in toddlers and preschool children with type 1 diabetes mellitus. J Pediatr. 2002;141:490–5.
McMahon SK, Airey FL, Marangou DA, et al. Insulin pump therapy in children and adolescents: improvements in key parameters of diabetes management including quality of life. Diabet Med. 2005;22:92–6.
Retnakaran R, Hochman J, DeVries JH, et al. Continuous subcutaneous insulin infusion versus multiple daily injections: the impact of baseline A1C. Diabetes Care. 2004;27:2590–6.
Pankowska E, Blazik M, Dziechciarz P, Szypowska A, Szajewska H. Continuous subcutaneous insulin infusion vs. multiple daily injections in children with type 1 diabetes: a systematic review and meta-analysis of randomized control trials. Pediatr Diabetes. 2009;10:52–8.
DiMeglio LA, Pottorff TM, Boyd SR, France L, Fineberg N, Eugster EA. A randomized, controlled study of insulin pump therapy in diabetic preschoolers. J Pediatr. 2004;145:380–4.
Fox LA, Buckloh LM, Smith SD, Wysocki T, Mauras N. A randomized controlled trial of insulin pump therapy in young children with type 1 diabetes. Diabetes Care. 2005;28:1277–81.
Churchill JN, Ruppe RL, Smaldone A. Use of continuous insulin infusion pumps in young children with type 1 diabetes: a systematic review. J Pediatr Health Care. 2009;23:173–9.
Weinzimer SA, Swan KL, Sikes KA, Ahern JH. Emerging evidence for the use of insulin pump therapy in infants, toddlers, and preschool-aged children with type 1 diabetes. Pediatr Diabetes. 2006;7(Suppl 4):15–9.
Forlenza GP, Buckingham B, Maahs DM. Progress in diabetes technology: developments in insulin pumps, continuous glucose monitors, and progress towards the artificial pancreas. J Pediatr. 2016;169:13–20.
Kowalski A. Pathway to artificial pancreas systems revisited: moving downstream. Diabetes Care. 2015;38:1036–43.

Ly TT, Layne JE, Huyett LM, Nazzaro D, O'Connor JB. Novel Bluetooth-enabled tubeless insulin pump: innovating pump therapy for patients in the digital age. J Diabetes Sci Technol. 2019;13:20–6.

Edelman SV, Bode BW, Bailey TS, et al. Insulin pump therapy in patients with type 2 diabetes safely improved glycemic control using a simple insulin dosing regimen. Diabetes Technol Ther. 2010;12:627–33.

Vigersky RA, Huang S, Cordero TL, et al., OpT2mise Study Group. Improved HbA1c, total daily insulin dose, and treatment satisfaction with insulin pump therapy compares to multiple daily injections in patients with type 2 diabetes irrespective of baseline C-peptide levels. Endocr Pract. 2018;24:446–52.

Aronson R, Reznik Y, Conget I, et al., OpT2mise Study Group. Sustained efficacy of insulin pump therapy compared with multiple daily injections in type 2 diabetes: 12-month data from the OpT2mise randomized trial. Diabetes Obes Metab. 2016;18:500–7.

Reznik Y, Cohen O, Aronson R, et al., OpT2mise Study Group. Insulin pump treatment compared with multiple daily injections for treatment of type 2 diabetes (OpT2mise): a randomised open-label controlled trial. Lancet. 2014;384:1265–72.

King AB, Clark D, Wolfe GS. The number of basal rates required to achieve near-normal basal glucose control in pump-treated type 2 diabetes. Diabetes Technol Ther. 2012;14:900–3.

Skyler JS, Ponder S, Kruger DM, Matheson D, Parkin CG. Is there a place for insulin pump therapy in your practice? Clin Diabetes. 2007;25:50–6.

Knutsen PG, Voelker CQ, Nikkel CC. Clinical insights into a new, disposable insulin delivery device. Diabetes Spectr. 2015;28:209–13.

Lilly LC, Mader JK, Warner J. Developing a simple 3-day insulin delivery device to meet the needs of people with type 2 diabetes. J Diabetes Sci Technol. 2019;13:11–9.

Hermanns N, Lilly LC, Mader JK, et al. Novel simple insulin delivery device reduces barriers to insulin therapy in type 2 diabetes: results from a pilot study. J Diabetes Sci Technol. 2015;9:581–7.

Mader JK, Lilly LC, Aberer F, et al. Improved glycaemic control and treatment satisfaction with a simple wearable 3-day insulin delivery device among people with type 2 diabetes. Diabet Med. 2018;35:1448–56.

Bergenstal RM, Tamborlane WV, Ahmann A, et al. Effectiveness of sensor-augmented insulin-pump therapy in type 1 diabetes. N Engl J Med. 2010;363:311–20.

Slover RH, Welsh JB, Criego A, et al. Effectiveness of sensor-augmented pump therapy in children and adolescents with type 1 diabetes in the STAR 3 study. Pediatr Diabetes. 2012;13:6–11.

Steineck I, Ranjan A, Norgaard K, Schmidt S. Sensor-augmented insulin pumps and hypoglycemia prevention in type 1 diabetes. J Diabetes Sci Technol. 2017;11:50–8.

DCCT/EDIC Research Group. Intensive diabetes treatment and cardiovascular outcomes in type 1 diabetes: the DCCT/EDIC Study 30-year follow-up. Diabetes Care. 2016;39:686–93.

Awoniyi O, Rehman R, Dagogo-Jack S. Hypoglycemia in patients with type 1 diabetes: epidemiology, pathogenesis, and prevention. Curr Diabetes Rep. 2013;13:669–78.

Bergenstal RM, Klonoff DC, Garg SK, et al. Threshold-based insulin-pump interruption for reduction of hypoglycemia. N Engl J Med. 2013;369:224–32.

Danne T, Kordonouri O, Holder M, et al. Prevention of hypoglycemia by using low glucose suspend function in sensor-augmented pump therapy. Diabetes Technol Ther. 2011;13:1129–34.

Maahs DM, Calhoun P, Buckingham BA, et al. A randomized trial of a home system to reduce nocturnal hypoglycemia in type 1 diabetes. Diabetes Care. 2014;37:1885–91.

Buckingham BA, Raghinaru D, Cameron F, et al. Predictive low-glucose insulin suspension reduces duration of nocturnal hypoglycemia in children without increasing ketosis. Diabetes Care. 2015;38:1197–204.

Forlenza GP, Li Z, Buckingham BA, et al. Predictive low-glucose suspend reduces hypoglycemia in adults, adolescents, and children with type 1 diabetes in an at-home randomized crossover study: results of the PROLOG Trial. Diabetes Care. 2018;41:2155–61.

Abraham MB, Nicholas JA, Smith GJ, et al. Reduction in hypoglycemia with the predictive low-glucose management system: a long-term randomized controlled trial in adolescents with type 1 diabetes. Diabetes Care. 2018;41:303–10.
Buckingham BA, Christiansen MP, Forlenza GP, et al. Performance of the Omnipod personalized model predictive control algorithm with meal bolus challenges in adults with type 1 diabetes. Diabetes Technol Ther. 2018;20:585–95.
Forlenza GP, Cameron FM, Ly TT, et al. Fully closed-loop multiple model probabilistic predictive controller artificial pancreas performance in adolescents and adults in a supervised hotel setting. Diabetes Technol Ther. 2018;20:335–43.
Zisser H, Renard E, Kovatchev B, et al. Multicenter closed-loop insulin delivery study points to challenges for keeping blood glucose in a safe range by a control algorithm in adults and adolescents with type 1 diabetes from various sites. Diabetes Technol Ther. 2014;16:613–22.
Buckingham BA, Forlenza GP, Pinsker JE, et al. Safety and feasibility of the OmniPod hybrid closed-loop system in adult, adolescent, and pediatric patients with type 1 diabetes using a personalized model predictive control algorithm. Diabetes Technol Ther. 2018;20:257–62.
Brown S, Raghinaru D, Emory E, Kovatchev B. First look at Control-IQ: a new-generation automated insulin delivery system. Diabetes Care. 2018;41:2634–6.
Weisman A, Bai JW, Cardinez M, Kramer CK, Perkins BA. Effect of artificial pancreas systems on glycaemic control in patients with type 1 diabetes: a systematic review and meta-analysis of outpatient randomised controlled trials. Lancet Diabetes Endocrinol. 2017;5:501–12.
Garg SK, Weinzimer SA, Tamborlane WV, et al. Glucose outcomes with the in-home use of a hybrid closed-loop insulin delivery system in adolescents and adults with type 1 diabetes. Diabetes Technol Ther. 2017;19:155–63.
Lewis D. History and perspective on DIY closed looping. J Diabetes Sci Technol. 2018; https://doi.org/10.1177/1932296818808307.
American Diabetes Association. Children and adolescents: standards of medical care in diabetes—2018. Diabetes Care. 2018;41(Suppl 1):S126–36.
Sherr JL, Tauschmann M, Battelino T, et al. ISPAD clinical practice consensus guidelines 2018: diabetes technologies. Pediatr Diabetes. 2018;19(Suppl 27):302–25.
Peters AL, Ahmann AJ, Battelino T, et al. Diabetes technology: continuous subcutaneous insulin infusion therapy and continuous glucose monitoring in adults: an Endocrine Society clinical practice guideline. J Clin Endocrinol Metab. 2016;101:3922–37.
Grunberger G, Handelsman Y, Bloomgarden ZT, et al. American Association of Clinical Endocrinologists and American College of Endocrinology 2018 position statement on integration of insulin pumps and continuous glucose monitoring in patients with diabetes mellitus. Endocr Pract. 2018;24:302–8.
Tanenbaum ML, Hanes SJ, Miller KM, Naranjo D, Bensen R, Hood KK. Diabetes device use in adults with type 1 diabetes: barriers to uptake and potential intervention targets. Diabetes Care. 2017;40:181–7.
Forlenza GP, Messer LH, Berget C, Wadwa RP, Driscoll KA. Biopsychosocial factors associated with satisfaction and sustained use of artificial pancreas technology and its components: a call to the technology field. Curr Diab Rep. 2018;18:114.
Rashotte J, Tousignant K, Richardson C, et al. Living with sensor-augmented pump therapy in type 1 diabetes: adolescents' and parents' search for harmony. Can J Diabetes. 2014;38:256–62.
Ritholz MD, Atakov-Castillo A, Beste M, et al. Psychosocial factors associated with use of continuous glucose monitoring. Diabetes Med. 2010;27:1060–5.
Messer LH, Johnson R, Driscoll KA, Jones J. Best friend or spy: a qualitative meta-synthesis on the impact of continuous glucose monitoring on life with type 1 diabetes. Diabetes Med. 2018;35:409–18.
Naranjo D, Suttiratana SC, Iturralde E, et al. What end users and stakeholders want from automated insulin delivery systems. Diabetes Care. 2017;40:1453–61.
Iturralde E, Tanenbaum ML, Hanes SJ, et al. Expectations and attitudes of individuals with type 1 diabetes after using a hybrid closed loop system. Diabetes Educ. 2017;43:223–32.

Messer LH, Berget C, Beatson C, Polsky S, Forlenza GP. Preserving skin integrity with chronic device use in diabetes. Diabetes Technol Ther. 2018;20(Suppl 2):S254–64.

Hofer SE, Heidtmann B, Raile K, et al. Discontinuation of insulin pump treatment in children, adolescents, and young adults: a multicenter analysis based on the DPV database in Germany and Austria. Pediatr Diabetes. 2010;11:116–21.

Low KG, Massa L, Lehman D, Olshan JS. Insulin pump use in young adolescents with type 1 diabetes: a descriptive study. Pediatr Diabetes. 2005;6:22–31.

Hirsch IB. Clinical review: realistic expectations and practical use of continuous glucose monitoring for the endocrinologist. J Clin Endocrinol Metab. 2009;94:2232–8.

Messer LH. Why expectations will determine the future of artificial pancreas. Diabetes Technol Ther. 2018;20(Suppl 2):S265–8.

Burdick J, Chase HP, Slover RH, et al. Missed insulin meal boluses and elevated hemoglobin A1c levels in children receiving insulin pump therapy. Pediatrics. 2004;113:e221–4.

Olinder AL, Kernell A, Smide B. Missed bolus doses: devastating for metabolic control in CSII-treated adolescents with type 1 diabetes. Pediatr Diabetes. 2009;10:142–8.

Patton SR, Driscoll KA, Clements MA. Adherence to insulin pump behaviors in young children with type 1 diabetes mellitus. J Diabetes Sci Technol. 2017;11:87–91.

Westen SC, Warnick JL, Albanese-O'Neill A, et al. Objectively measured adherence in adolescents with type 1 diabetes on multiple daily injections and insulin pump therapy. J Pediatr Psychol. 2019;44:21–31.

Hood KK, Peterson CM, Rohan JM, Drotar D. Association between adherence and glycemic control in pediatric type 1 diabetes: a meta-analysis. Pediatrics. 2009;124:e1171–9.

American Association of Diabetes Educators. AADE practice paper: continuous subcutaneous insulin infusion (CSII) without and with sensor integration. Diabetes Educ. 2018;44(3 Suppl):S32–53.

Heinemann L, Fleming GA, Petrie JR, Holl RW, Bergenstal RM, Peters AL. Insulin pump risks and benefits: a clinical appraisal of pump safety standards, adverse event reporting and research needs. A joint statement of the European Association for the Study of Diabetes and the American Diabetes Association Diabetes Technology Working Group. Diabetologia. 2015;58(5):862–70.

Berget C, Thomas SE, Messer L, Beatson C, Polsky S, Forlenza GP. A clinical training program for hybrid closed loop therapy in a pediatric diabetes clinic. J Diabetes Sci Technol. 2019;13(4):745–53.

Chapter 6
Algorithmic Automated Insulin Dosing

Julia Schulman-Bergen

Advances in insulin pump technology including automated insulin delivery (AID) systems have been life-changing for people living with diabetes (PwD). These systems have been shown to increase patient time in range (TIR), minimize hypoglycemia, and decrease the burden of diabetes for individuals living with diabetes. AID systems integrate an insulin pump with a continuous glucose monitoring system and utilize a control algorithm which adjusts insulin delivery in response to real-time sensor glucose levels, rates of change, meal intake, and other factors including active insulin times. Unlike a truly "artificial pancreas" these systems still require users to manually program insulin boluses with meals and thus are also referred to as Hybrid Closed Loop (HCL) insulin pumps.

As a person living with diabetes for over 20 years I have firsthand knowledge of the burden of type 1 diabetes. For many years, I anxiously awaited the approval of an AID system and dreamt of a time when I would be able to maintain tight glucose control without the constant mental burden of adjusting doses, measuring the food I ate, how active I was, how much mental stress I was under in addition to other many other factors which are constantly affecting blood glucose. While my own type 1 diabetes is still something that requires daily management, the constant feeling of micro-managing all aspects of my life due to my diabetes, no longer looms over me. While AIDs (Automated Insulin Delivery) are certainly not a magical cure for type 1 diabetes, many PwD express a significant decrease in the burden of diabetes when switching to an AID.

J. Schulman-Bergen (✉)
Medicine Service Line, Northwell Health, Floral Park, NY, USA
e-mail: JSchulman@northwell.edu

S. Fishman (ed.), *Advances in Diabetes Technology*, Contemporary Endocrinology, https://doi.org/10.1007/978-3-031-75352-7_6

Advancements in Technology and the Development of Automated Insulin Delivery Systems

The concept of glucose-responsive insulin delivery has been studied for many years but the lack of a reliable and accurate CGM (Continuous Glucose Monitoring), limitations in insulin pump device connectivity, and insulin action profiles have delayed development of true closed loop insulin pumps [1].

The first iterations of glucose-responsive insulin delivery were developed in the 1960s and 1970 using venous glucose measurements to control intravenous infusion of insulin and dextrose to help maintain euglycemia. These devices, fashioned from chemotherapy infusion devices, were used while patients were admitted to the hospital, were only for clinical research, and were far from comfortable for patients to wear for regular insulin delivery. Over the past 60 years, these cumbersome devices have transformed into pager-sized wearable devices with connectivity to glucose sensors and smart phones. These advances have allowed PwDs (Patients with type 1 diabetes) to leave behind some of the disease burden that can be so overwhelming [1].

The precursor to HCL systems, sensor-augmented pumps (SAP) were developed in the 2000s when significant advances in glucose sensor technology and improved insurance coverage allowed for more widespread use of CGMS. These original SAPs (Sensor-Augmented Pumps) allowed PwDs the ability to link their sensor directly to their pump with the glucose displayed on the screen of their Insulin Pump [2]. Once connectivity between sensor and pump was established, further innovation came quickly with the development of the earliest automated insulin delivery device which included a low glucose suspend feature. These systems suspended insulin delivery once the CGM crossed a specific glucose threshold [1, 3]. While these systems decreased the amount and severity of hypoglycemia, this was at times at the expense of rebound hyperglycemia. Unlike current sensors, these devices did not predict glucose levels in the future, so insulin was often suspended too late to prevent all episodes of hypoglycemia. These systems were not designed to deliver additional insulin based on elevated sensor glucose so did nothing to prevent hyperglycemia. Despite this barrier, low glucose suspend pumps were widely adopted by PwDs with great excitement as the reduction of hypoglycemia was a considerable benefit. Many patients reported significant decreases in hypoglycemic-related anxiety and reported improvement in sleep and quality of life once utilizing these new systems [4].

Algorithms and Hybrid Closed Loop Systems

Currently available AID algorithms have been developed using three different algorithmic concepts—proportional-integral-derivative (PID) control, model predictive control (MPC), and fuzzy logic knowledge-based systems [2, 5, 6]. These algorithms are the backbone to our AID systems and calculate insulin infusion as a function of time and changing glucose concentration. Each algorithm utilizes different parameters for insulin action time, carbohydrate intake, insulin sensitivity, and other factors and thus offers different benefits for people living with diabetes.

PID Control Algorithms

PID systems, often used in control engineering, are the simplest of our current algorithms and utilize calculations of the individual component (P—proportional, i—integral, d—derivative). This mathematical model predicts how the system will behave in the future and uses this prediction to determine the best control inputs to achieve the desired outcomes.

In the case of insulin pumps, the PID algorithm uses real-time information considering the proportional factor of how far sensor glucose is from the set target, the integral factor of how long sensor glucose has been away from the target and the derivative factor of how rapidly the sensor glucose has been changing [2, 5].

Model Predictive Control Algorithms

Model Predictive Control (MPC) is a control algorithm which utilizes a mathematical model to predict future behavior and optimize control actions to achieve the desired objective. The model predictive control algorithm first predicts the system's future behavior and then uses those predictions, helping determine the best control actions needed to achieve the desired outcome. This system delivers insulin based on glucose values expected as determined by the rtCGMS. When an insulin bolus (termed micro bolus in adaptive basal insulin delivery) is administered, the system calculates future glucose values based on current glucose levels and insulin on board (IOB). When the calculated glucose levels are within the desired range the system will deliver the micro bolus. When calculated glucose concentrations are higher or lower than targeted values, the doses will be increased or decreased based on these values [2, 6].

Fuzzy Logic Control (FLC)

Fuzzy logic control algorithms utilize a set of rules based on fuzzy logic, a form of mathematical reasoning that allows for uncertainty and imprecision in the input and output. These algorithms are based on fuzzy set theory, which allows for more flexible and approximate reasoning compared to traditional binary logic. Within an insulin pump framework, fuzzy logic considers sensor glucose predictions, meal information, and activity levels to determine appropriate insulin dosing [2, 6].

Currently Available HCL Systems in United States

Medtronic 670g/770g

The PID control algorithm was used to develop the Medtronic MiniMed 670g system, the first commercial AID to receive regulatory approval in the United States. As the first system to gain regulatory approvals, the system was anticipated with great excitement by the diabetes community. The 770g system, MiniMed's most recently released CSII utilizes this same algorithm as the 670g with some updated components. Both systems utilize Medtronic's own sensor, the Guardian 3 CGMS. The system is approved only for people with type 1 diabetes aged 2 and above.

One common and significant concern with the MiniMed system care the calibration reminders that the system requires to stay in automode. While using the MiniMed 670g/770g in automode, calibrations of the Guardian 3 CGMS are still required. This is in stark contrast to the two other commercially available systems which utilize a sensor that requires no user calibration. In response to frustrations with the 670g system, updates to the 770g helped increase the average time spent in automode from 80.5% to 87.5% by improving sensor connectivity and decreasing calibrations needed [6].

Despite these improvements, the Guardian 3 CGMS still requires calibrations every 12 h at a minimum during its 7-day wear and on the first day of sensor wear calibrations must also occur within the first 2 h of wear and again within 6 h [6]. For patients looking to minimize the burden of diabetes by switching to an AID device, this need to frequently test glucose can be disappointing and frustrating. Additional alerts can continue throughout sensor wear. The PwD may receive a "calibrate now" alert if the system detects sensory accuracy concerns. Many patients report significant frustration with the interruptions these frequent alerts cause in daily life.

The Medtronic 670g/770g System Operates in Three Modes: Automode, Manual Mode, and Safe Basal

While in automode, basal insulin (termed auto basal in this HCL system) is delivered based on a PwDs sensor glucose values and recent insulin delivery. The MiniMed 670g and 770g has a pre-set target of 120 mg/dL and the algorithm uses micro boluses every 5 min to attempt to maintain glucose levels at this set target. During periods with increased exercise, while patients are NPO or during occurrences when a higher target might be desirable, the patient can set a temporary target value of 150 mg/dL to decrease the risk of hypoglycemia.

Unlike other AIDs on the market, the MiniMed AID system must be operated in manual mode for at least 48 h prior to activating automation as the system must first analyze patients TDD (Total Daily Dose) before system adjustments can begin [6]. During automode delivery, the MiniMed CSII receives a glucose value from the rtCGM every 5 min. Based on this rtCGMS data, the system can calculate a correction micro bolus based on current glucose, target glucose, insulin sensitivity factor, how long the insulin remains active in the PwD and how much active insulin is still working in the PwD. Sensitivity is calculated in the 670g by averaging the total daily dose (TDD) of the last 6 days and applying the 1800 rule where insulin sensitivity factor is equivalent to 1800 divided by a patient's total daily dose [6].

An additional mode in the 670g/770g is safe basal which occurs when a patient's pump is in automode, but it is not adjusting the systems basal based on the sensor glucose readings. While in safe basal mode, the system uses the recent insulin delivery to automatically deliver a fixed rate of basal insulin. Sensor glucose values are not used to determine the automatic basal rates [6].

Safe basal mode can occur for several reasons including when a senor glucose reading is not available due to communication issues, sensor calibration expiring, during sensor warm-up, when blood glucose is different from sensor glucose by 35% or more, or when automode has been at personal minimum automode basal for 2½ h or maximum automode basal for 4 h. The system will stay in safe basal for up to 90 min. If the situation is resolved, the pump will revert to automode, if not, it will continue basal insulin deliver in manual mode [6].

Like stand-alone insulin pumps, the insulin to carbohydrate ratio (or how many grams of carbohydrate are covered by 1 unit of insulin) determines the insulin that will be delivered for the meal portion of the bolus. The PwD enters the amount of carbohydrates in grams into the system, and the pump will suggest a bolus based on this input. The user can enter up to eight different insulin to carbohydrate factors for use throughout the day. This carbohydrate factor will also affect the basal insulin delivery as frequent or inadequate boluses will change the PwD TDD and the patient's insulin sensitivity factor, which is redetermined by the system each day at midnight [6].

This system allows for providers or PwD to modify two parameters while using the pump in automated mode: Insulin Action Time (IAT) and carbohydrate ratio. Adjusting a patient's basal insulin rates or insulin sensitivity while using this system will not alter insulin delivery while the system is in automode. When adjusting settings, the provider should remember that if insulin action time is set to a shorter time, the micro bolus being delivered will be larger.

As the first HCL system to receive Food and Drug Administration clearance, the MiniMed has many pre-set safety features. The algorithm will only allow for 2.5 times the average basal insulin amount to be delivered during the day to prevent over-delivery of insulin due to regulatory precautions created by the Food and Drug Administration. PwD who utilize post-prandial dosing of mealtime insulin rather than pre-prandial will often notice hyperglycemia following meals that may not be corrected properly due to this basal maximum. Therefore, it is of utmost importance that boluses are provided prior to mealtime to avoid large post-prandial excursions. A correction bolus can be administered as a back-up if the PID algorithm does not reach target due to the maximum basal delivery being reached. The AID will recommend a correction dose to bring glucose to 150 mg/dL and further adjustment to the target of 120 mg/dL is then performed by the PID algorithm.

Medtronic's 780g, expected to launch in 2023 will offer an advanced closed loop allowing for a setpoint with a lower glucose target of 100–120 mg/dL and deliver 100% correction to meet target. Corrections will be delivered every 5 min as needed. Their eventual goal of a personalized closed loop will allow for optional carbohydrate counting, adapt with behavior and physiology and improved connectivity through smart phone control. Their 780g will continue to require 1 calibration on day 1 only but will require no further calibrations for the remainder of sensor weartime [6].

T:slim X2 Control IQ

The Tandem t:slim X2 Control-IQ (CIQ) system utilizes the Model Predictive Control (MPC) algorithm and combines the t:slim X2 insulin pump, the Dexcom G6 CGMS, and control IQ HCL control algorithm [7]. Control IQ technology adjusts insulin delivery rates in response to CGMS values and has three distinct modes; control IQ technology, sleep activity, and exercise mode. The target CGM ranges are not customizable with this system and vary depending on which mode the system is in. The system will remain operating in control IQ mode unless the sensor is in warm-up and will revert to manual mode if there is no sensor data for >20 min. Control IQ should not be used by anyone under 6 years old, in patients using less than 10 units of insulin/day or weighing less than 55 pounds [8].

During the system's initial setup, the clinical provider will input an individualized personal profile which includes the patient's basal rates, insulin carbohydrate ratio, and sensitivity. While using the system in control IQ mode, the target glucose and active insulin time are not customizable. The target glucose will be determined based on which mode the system is set to. Control IQ mode is designed to maintain a PwDs active personal profile settings when glucose levels are between 112.5 and 160 mg/dL. While in sleep mode the system will maintain the active personal profile when glucose is between 112.5 and 120 mg/dL and in exercise mode when glucose is between 140 and 160 mg/dL. While in control IQ technology and exercise mode, the system will deliver an automatic correction bolus if sensor glucose is predicted to be above 180 mg/dL within the next 30 min [8]. Automatic correction boluses are not delivered during sleep mode to help prevent hypoglycemia while patients are asleep.

The system will increase basal insulin delivery in control IQ mode when glucose is above 160 mg/dL, in sleep mode when glucose is above 120 mg/dL and in exercise mode when glucose is above 160 mg/dL. To prevent hypoglycemia, in control

IQ technology and sleep activity the system will decrease basal with glucose predicted to be below 112.5 and stop basal if glucose is predicted to be below 70 mg/dL. Bolus delivery is still possible even when basal delivery is suspended. In exercise mode, basal rate will be decreased when glucose is below 140 mg/dL and suspended with glucose below 80 mg/dL for additional protection from low glucose.

Automated correction boluses are available within this system but are designed to be modest to help improve elevated glucose while preventing hypoglycemia. The system will deliver the correction dose up to 60% of the calculated correction bolus once per hour as needed. The target glucose for automatic correction bolus is set at 110 mg/dL and is not adjustable. Automatic correction boluses will not be delivered within 60 min of the start, cancellation, or completion of an automatic or manual bolus to prevent stacking of insulin [8].

As with all HCL systems, bolusing prior to the meal is important to prevent postprandial elevations in glucose. The recent addition of a remote bolus feature allows patients the choice of bolusing for meal either from the on body pump or from the t-connect mobile app on compatible smart phones and should help in adherence with mealtime boluses.

While in sleep mode, the t-slim does not provide automatic correction boluses but adjusts insulin to a tighter glucose target using basal modulation. Automatic correction boluses may be more helpful in certain instances including missed boluses when compared to basal modulation so providers should determine if sleep mode provides a benefit for individual patients. Patients who often skip boluses later in the night might see better glucose control overnight if the system is kept in control IQ mode. Starting sleep mode 1–2 h after the last meal or snack and stopping sleep at least an hour prior to waking can be helpful to patients noticing significant hyperglycemia. Patients may benefit from turning off sleep mode completely during times of high stress, growth spurts, or steroid use [8].

Exercise mode, which sets target glucose levels at a higher number, should be considered for patients during times patients have greater risk for hypoglycemia. Exercise mode is appropriate to use for patients following increased alcohol consumption, while intermittent fasting, when NPO for medical procedures, during episodes of nausea or vomiting, for patients with hypoglycemic unawareness or fear of hypoglycemia, and elderly patients at higher risk for hypoglycemia.

Since the control IQ algorithm adjusts basal rate from patients pre-set personal profiles, when rapid changes in insulin requirements occur, patients may require an alternate personal profile. Patients can personalize up to six profiles and my find additional profiles beneficial for rapid changes in insulin demands such as when the patient is experiencing hyperglycemia secondary to steroid use or due to hormonal changes due to menstrual cycles [8].

Model Predictive Control and the Omnipod 5

The Omnipod 5 is the only fully on body Automated Insulin Delivery system available and utilizes a model predictive algorithm built into each POD. For patients looking for a tube-free AID system, the approval of the Omnipod 5 in 2022 was widely anticipated. While using the system in its automated version, the Dexcom g6 CGM transmits CGM data directly to the POD every 5 min thus allowing the PwD to have full on body insulin automation even when the controller is not within range of the POD. The Omnipod 5 is fully operated using either a compatible smartphone or a stand-alone controller supplied by the manufacturer. The controller does need to be present for bolus delivery and for the user to receive notifications [9].

The imbedded AID algorithm termed SmartAdjust technology is guided by total daily insulin delivery tracking to determine an "adaptive basal rate" as the baseline for adjusting insulin delivery. When first starting the system, the total daily dose is estimated based on the pre-programmed basal rates allowing the system to enter automated mode immediately from the start of use. Once wearing the system, PwD are not able to adjust basal rates as the system continually adapts these rates based on system history and the current CGM value and trend [9].

During the first POD wear, the SmartAdjust technology will track TDD and begins using this value to automate insulin delivery with future PODs. This TDD is updated with each POD change allowing for changes in insulin delivery as patients' needs change. This is especially important in the pediatric population as puberty and growth spurts lead to frequent changes in basal requirements. In addition to this learnt adaptivity, the system can also automatically increase, decrease, or pause delivery at any time to protect against hypoglycemia and hyperglycemia and will always pause delivery with glucose levels below 60 mg/dL [10].

Unlike other available AID systems, the Omnipod 5 system allows for a patient to select a glucose target between 110 and 150 mg/dL in 10 mg/dL increments. Different targets can be customized for various times of day. In general, a lower target usually equates to more TIR and lower mean glucose, whereas a higher target equates to less TIR, higher mean glucose, and reduced hypoglycemia risk [11].

The Omnipod 5 utilizes a programmable activity feature which will temporarily change the targeted glucose to 150 mg/dL during periods where hypoglycemia is of greater concern [10]. The activity feature was designed with aerobic exercise in mind but can also be used for alcohol use, time away from caregivers, or while patients are NPO.

Unique to the Omnipod 5 system is POD adaptivity. During the first POD wear or following a long break in wearing the system, the Omnipod 5 system will use the pre-programmed basal rate from manual mode as a starting point to adjust a PwDs insulin. After 48 h of the system collecting data, SmartAdjust technology stops adjusting insulin based on the pre-programmed active basal setting and starts using the adaptive basal rate for automated basal rate for subsequent POD changes [9].

This adaptive basal rate changes over time to best meet the PwD current insulin needs. The last 4–5 pods have the greatest effect with a decaying total daily insulin amount dictating the basal insulin delivery [9]. While the adaptive rate serves as a baseline, SmartAdjust technology will increase, decrease, or pause insulin to help maintain glucose at target levels alleviating the need for the clinician to finetune basal rates overtime.

While the Omnipod 5 system is in automated mode, it is still essential that patient's bolus prior to meals. Although the systems algorithm will increase insulin delivery with rising glucose levels, the automated response is not sufficient to fully counter post-meal glucose excursions. The SmartBolus calculator embedded in the Omnipod 5 calculates a suggested bolus, much like other bolus calculators, based on glucose, carbohydrate intake, and a pre-set insulin to carbohydrate ratio and insulin sensitivity rate. Unique to this system, the bolus calculator will also consider the trend of the CGM values. While CGMS values are trending up, the smart bolus calculator will try to keep glucose within range by adding up to 30% more insulin to the correction bolus. When CGMS data shows values trending downwards the smart bolus calculator will subtract up to 100% of the suggested insulin from the correction bolus. While glucose levels remain steady, the smart bolus calculator will offer no adjustment to the calculated correction bolus. Patients can accept or change any recommendations offered by the system and may make these changes due to anticipated activity, alcohol consumption, or other variables [9].

As previously mentioned, the Omnipod 5 system reduces and/or suspends insulin delivery if glucose is trending down or below target, resulting in little IOB leading up to mealtimes. As a result, many individuals may need stronger ICRs with AID therapy compared with nonautomated insulin delivery regimens [12].

As with all HCL systems, parameters that affect system performance include basal program, target glucose, insulin to carbohydrate ratio, correction factor, and duration of insulin action. The target glucose dictates target for automated delivery and informs all user-initiated boluses so when patients are noticing high or low glucose in between meals this is a good parameter to adjust. The insulin to carbohydrate and correction factor can be adjusted while in automated mode and is used to inform all user-initiated boluses. While the duration of insulin action is used for all user-initiated boluses, it does not affect automated delivery [9].

A patient's POD and CGMS can lose connection while in automated mode for several reasons including environmental interference, sensor-warm up or POD and CGMS not being within line of sight on the patient's body. When this occurs, SmartAdjust technology can no longer fully adjust insulin delivery. After 20 min of the POD not receiving data from the CGMS, the system will transition to "limited mode." While in limited mode, the device will never give more than the basal program active during manual mode. The system will automatically revert to automatic mode once the sensor and POD are communicating again. SmartAdjust technology is approved for anyone above the age of 2 years old and should not be used in patients taking less than 5 units of insulin per day. This technology is not approved in pregnant patients or those on dialysis [9].

The CARES Framework

The CARES framework was designed by researchers to better understand the difference of the various AID systems and utilizes a 5-step framework to compare currently available systems to help patients and caregivers choose the right AID for themselves or their patients. The framework compares how each system *calculates* insulin delivery, which parameters can be *adjusted*, when users will *revert* to traditional insulin pump settings, critical *education* points and key aspects of the *sensor and sharing* capabilities of the system. This clinical framework can guide clinicians in different clinical rules that apply to each system without requiring them to have proficiency in the algorithmic nuances of each device as the paradigm highlights fundamental components which have clinical relevance [13]. In general, patients should be given a choice in determining which AID system is the best fit for their diabetes.

Benefits of Automated Insulin Delivery Systems

Automated insulin delivery systems have been proven to improve time in range, reduce the frequency of hypoglycemic events, reduce risks of Diabetic Ketoacidosis (DKA), and improve quality of life for PwD.

As a person living with diabetes, the burden of the disease can be consuming. On a normal day, patients must monitor every piece of food eaten, perform dose calculations, monitor glucose, and account for activity levels and stress in addition to all of life's other demands. Even the most educated and insightful patients with deep understanding of the disease process will struggle with hypoglycemia and hyperglycemia regularly. This burden of diabetes can lead to considerable anxiety and depression for patients and fear of hypoglycemia can negatively impact patients' sleep. Avoidance of hypoglycemia due to these fears can lead to uncontrolled diabetes and significant long-term complications. The use of automated insulin devices can reduce the burden of diabetes management by simplifying insulin dosing and reducing the need for frequent glucose monitoring. In a survey of adults with type 1 diabetes, participants reported a significant reduction in diabetes-related distress and improved quality of life after using a closed loop system for 6 months [14].

Improved sleep quality has also been reported with the use of AID systems and many patients with diabetes notice this as one of the most significant improvements in quality of life when beginning AID therapy. Studies have shown that AIDs can improve sleep quality by reducing the need for overnight glucose monitoring and the risk of nocturnal hypoglycemia. In a study involving adults with type 1 diabetes, the use of a HCL insulin pump resulted in a significant reduction in the number of overnight glucose checks and a significant improvement in sleep quality compared to sensor-augmented pump therapy [15].

Randomized clinical trials have demonstrated a clear superiority of HCL systems compared to stand-alone CSII and MDI with and without CGMS. Studies demonstrated improvement in hemoglobin A1c, reduction of both hyperglycemic and hypoglycemic events, and improved time in range. HCL systems have demonstrated the most improvement in glucose control during overnight periods when a reduction in extraneous factors like carbohydrate intake and exercise are minimized [16]. In a randomized controlled trial involving adults with type 1 diabetes, the use of a closed loop system resulted in a significant reduction in time spent in hypoglycemia and improved overall glucose control compared to a sensor-augmented pump therapy [17]. Findings from a retrospective analysis of 136 adult patients with type 1 diabetes demonstrated consistently improved results of euglycemia, lower glucose variability, and a reduction in hypoglycemic risk when comparing hybrid closed loop systems with sensor-augmented pump therapy and use of predictive low glucose algorithms. When researchers examined time in range with these different systems, the results were impressive for the hybrid closed loop systems. Participants in the HCL group spent more than 70% of their TIR compared with 32.7% in the PLGS group and 20.2% in the SAP cohort [18, 19].

The improvement in glycemic outcomes using AID systems has also been documented in children and adolescents. Researchers have observed the psychosocial benefits of AID systems in children ages 12–15 and observed psychological status of the study subjects by using a standard measurement tool called the Pediatric Quality of Life Inventory (PedsQL), a 23-item health status questionnaire used by both parent and child that evaluates physical functioning, emotional functioning, psychosocial functioning, social functioning, and school functioning in children ages 2–18. This research demonstrated "improved diabetes-specific quality of life" for children wearing AID system [20].

Challenges and Limitation of Automated Insulin Delivery Systems

As engineers and health care professionals have developed automated insulin delivery models, many barriers have stood in the way of creating a closed loop insulin pump. Issues with sensor accuracy, slow insulin action profiles, and different utilization of insulin during exercise continue to be of greatest concerns for future developments in insulin delivery. A true closed loop insulin pump would require no input from the patient regarding meal timing and amounts, changes in exercise levels, and other daily life variables and is still many years away from being available for the general population.

While accuracy of glucose sensors has improved over the years, glucose diffusion in the interstitial fluid of cells continues to delay glucose measured by rtCGMS systems compared to changes in blood glucose (BG), and this creates challenges in adjusting insulin based on sensor glucose values. Sensor accuracy is measured by

MARD or Mean Absolute Relative Difference, calculated by taking the absolute differences between the CGM value and referenced blood glucose values. The MARD is an important measure for assessing the performance of glucose sensors as it considers both the accuracy and precision of the sensor reading. Our currently available CGMS being utilized by AID systems have a MARD below 10% and thus have accuracy considered acceptable for guiding insulin therapy and diabetes management decisions.

Another significant factor delaying advances in system development is the action of currently available insulins. With insulin pumps utilizing exogenous insulin, patients see a delay in the absorption of insulin as it travels from the subcutaneous layer into the bloodstream. Exogenous insulin will first act in the periphery, rather than the liver, and this delay in suppressing hepatic glucose further slows the insulin's action. This delay creates an additional hurdle for developers as our currently available ultra-rapid-acting insulins action profiles are truly not that rapid. Our fastest insulins, Lyumjev and Fiasp, tend to have onset of action 20 min post dose, about 10 min faster when compared to Novolog or Humalog. During the first 30 min post dose, Lyumjev and Fiasp had a threefold greater glucose-lowering effect compared to Humalog and Novolog. Maximum glucose-lowering effect of Lyumjev and Fiasp occurs between 1 and 3 h after injection [21].

Candidate Selection for HCL

Many clinical providers still focus on "proper clinical selection" prior to starting patients on new diabetes technology despite the demonstrated significant and sustained glycemic improvements seen with AID systems. Currently no evidence-based criteria have been developed for beginning HCL systems. Some clinicians use personally created guidelines to select patients, and this decreases the number of patients being started on more advanced diabetes technology. The criteria providers use may include patients monitoring glucose a specific number of times per day, minimum number of patient visits per year, minimum duration of diabetes or specific A1c targets. Many of these criteria were important in the past when using stand-alone CSII but should be reevaluated with our newer technology.

For all patients utilizing insulin pumps, early detection of diabetic ketoacidosis is critical. Historically, there has been concern regarding increased risk of diabetic ketoacidosis (DKA) in patients managed on continuous insulin infusion devices due to concerns of occlusions preventing basal delivery. Despite these concerns, recent studies show a 0.84 reduced odd of diabetic ketoacidosis among insulin pump users compared to those managed on multiple daily injections [11]. While patient education on ketoacidosis is important prior to starting on a HCL system, the same would certainly be true for patients managed on MDI. Patients should be taught to check ketone levels when glucose levels remain elevated and do not respond to correction doses. The incorporation of CGMS into our insulin pumps may help to provide additional support to patients in preventing DKA as patients receive notifications that glucose levels are elevated and hopefully are trained to check for ketones during these instances.

The concept of patients needing SMBG frequently as a prerequisite to HCL systems is counterintuitive as current systems incorporate CGMS which are often approved to completely replace standard fingersticks. Patients should be trained to check fingersticks though anytime they notice a discrepancy in their sensor glucose readings versus any active symptoms to confirm accuracy of sensor.

In the past, many providers found it important for patients to have diabetes for a minimum amount of time before beginning CSII therapy. Rather than designate a time for having diabetes prior to starting therapy, basic diabetes knowledge would be a better prerequisite for beginning any diabetes technology. All patients with type 1 diabetes should understand how to check for and treat ketoacidosis and understand signs and symptoms of hypoglycemia and treatment. Carbohydrate counting should also be a prerequisite prior to starting a HCL as input of carbohydrate amount and glucose level prior to meals is hallmark to success on these systems.

Previously some providers would not allow patients with vastly uncontrolled glucose to begin CSII therapy, due to concern for Diabetic Ketoacidosis. Despite this, risk for ketoacidosis remains lower for patients managed on CSII and current patients with uncontrolled glucose have seen considerable improvement in control while switching to these devices.

If the PwD is trainable on the system and can demonstrate competency when being trained, there should be no reason to prevent patients from beginning therapy due to the number of visits per year, time since diagnosis or based on number of fingersticks daily. Current systems are user friendly and if a patient is competent enough to utilize a smart phone, they should be able to be trained on a AID system.

This non-evidence-based criteria for selecting potential insulin pump users may lead to disparities in diabetes technology among racial and ethnic minorities and are based on outdated viewpoints of CSII. Lower socioeconomic status, use of government-sponsored insurance and minority racial-ethnic status have been linked with higher A1c levels and lower use of technology including insulin pumps and sensors [11]. Providers should understand the many benefits of AID therapy and should recommend therapy to all patients with diabetes who can demonstrate competence when trained.

Do-It Yourself Closed Loop Systems

Unlike traditional insulin pumps which are proprietary and closed-source, open-source insulin pumps are designed to be open and transparent, with the software and hardware specifications freely available to users and developers. In 2013, due to frustration with the slow process of medical device development, concerns over the prohibitive cost of proprietary insulin pumps and a desire to have greater customization over devices, the #WeAreNotWaiting movement was born. This movement, started by PwD and their loved ones, encourages the sharing of information and open-source development and thereby accelerates the pace of innovation toward new and improved diabetes treatments [22].

The OpenAPS, or Open Artificial Pancreas System project, develops and applies open-access closed loop systems and created the first homemade artificial pancreas utilizing the oref0 (OpenAPS reference design zero) algorithm. This heuristic-based algorithm is designed to follow the same math a person with diabetes uses to make decisions about insulin adjustments and did not receive regulatory overview or approval. OpenAPS is designed to use existing approved medical devices, commodity hardware, and open-source software and requires a Do-It-Yourself implementation. PwDs can obtain documentation and advice from a community of people who have implemented the system themselves but must be willing to build their own system [22].

As of July 5, 2022, there are more than 2720+ individuals around the world using several types of DIY closed loop implementations. Observational before and after studies show improvements in TIR, HbA1c, and quality of life [22] but given these devices are not FDA (Food and Drug Administration) approved it is difficult to provide guidance to our patients when they may experience issues with these systems.

Ensuring Realistic Expectations

Setting realistic expectations before initiating any AID therapy is of utmost importance when beginning an AID system. Many individuals may expect an AID system to be a magical cure for their diabetes or for it to take over all control of their insulin delivery. This is not a realistic expectation of any of the currently available AID systems. Unrealistic expectations of these devices can increase the risk of user dissatisfaction and therapy discontinuation. For all patients' appropriate initial settings based on body weight, physiology and clinical needs of the user are key.

Patients starting these devices must know they will need to wear their CGMS and pump continuously to maximize time in automated modes. Bolusing prior to meals continues to be a hallmark of patient success on these systems. Common issues related to infusion sites, skin irritation, and pump malfunction that occur in standalone systems continue to be a potential barrier to success in AIDs (Automated Insulin Delivery) systems, but diabetes educators can assist patients in determining the best skin barriers or preparations for success.

While people with diabetes should understand that overall glycemia will improve when transitioning to an AID system, these systems will not eliminate all hypoglycemic and hyperglycemic excursions. Patients will still be required to change cartridges; infusion sets or PODs based on manufacturer guidance. Therefore, it is best to conceptualize AID as a tool to help improve diabetes management and reduce self-care burden, not as a means of eliminating the need for diabetes self-care.

Patient trust in the system is also important in a successful transition. While patients need to understand when to intervene with manual boluses, they must also learn to trust the system when using an AID. Some PwD who are accustomed to tightly controlling their own insulin delivery may find the transition to AIDs difficult. Patients should receive reassurance that the algorithm has been rigorously tested and was found to safely deliver insulin based on current glucose values and trends, while also considering factors such as IOB and patient-specific parameters [23]. When patients micro-manage their insulin delivery, they may lead to issues with the algorithm properly adjusting doses. Due to basal rates suspending at times, patients may want to consider treating low glucose levels with less carbohydrates (5–10 g) if insulin has been suspended prior to the low to prevent rebound hyperglycemia.

Dual Hormone Closed Loop Systems

While HCL has already been shown to be extremely valuable to those living with diabetes, barriers still exist in creating a true closed loop system. One of the most significant issues facing our current systems is the ability of our rapid-acting insulins to work quickly enough to prevent post-prandial elevations.

Dual hormone closed loop systems are being investigated to help address this issue and include systems that utilize either pramlintide or glucagon. When compared to single hormone HCL, dual hormone systems have shown a slightly lower time in hypoglycemia. No differences in the time in the target range have been identified [24].

Glucagon was first explored in the mid-2000s as an adjunct to insulin in closed loop systems to help prevent hypoglycemia. Even with insulin suspension, hypoglycemia can still occur in AID systems due to the slow onset and offset of short-acting insulin and the dysregulation of glucagon that occurs in type 1 diabetes. Dual hormone insulin-glucagon systems have been designed in two ways. The first utilizes small boluses of glucagon to prevent hypoglycemia and does not change insulin delivery. The second uses intermittent glucagon delivery and allows for more aggressive insulin delivery with the outcome of a lower glucose target [25].

Until recently, researchers were limited in creation of a real-world dual hormone insulin-glucagon system due to the stability of lyophilized glucagon preparations which needed to be reconstituted every 24 h. Now, several liquid stable glucagon products have gained FDA (Food and Drug Administration) approval allowing them to remain stable in a pump cartridge for greater than 24 h. While the safety of long-term glucagon dosing has been demonstrated in animals, this still needs to be established in humans [25] prior to widespread use of these systems.

The iLet, a dual hormone insulin-glucagon system commercially developed by Beta Bionics, improved hypoglycemia compared to a single hormone AID when exercise was announced 20 min prior to exercise. While comparisons between single hormone and dual hormone AIDs have been exploratory only, studies have shown time in range for both symptoms to be quite similar. There was a slight decrease in hypoglycemia in dual hormone insulin-glucagon systems but a tradeoff of slightly more hyperglycemia was seen [26].

Pramlintide, a synthetic derivative analog of amylin, is also being explored in dual hormone systems. In healthy individuals without type 1 diabetes, amylin is co-secreted with insulin by the pancreas and can have effects on delay of gastric emptying, which can be abnormally rapid in diabetes; suppression of glucagon and development of satiety shortly after starting to eat. When used with insulin, these effects limit post-meal hyperglycemia and prevent calorie intake [11]. Despite these benefits, Pramlintide use in type 1 diabetes is not common as it requires an additional injection with each meal and patients often report significant GI side effects [21]. Dual hormone HCL systems using pramlintide have been developed and studied but evidence is limited and has shown mixed results in patients' time in range [3, 26].

Fully Closed Loop Systems

Automated insulin delivery systems are rapidly evolving with new advances in AID systems occurring regularly. While currently available hybrid closed loop systems have revolutionized diabetes management for PwD, these systems still require patients to input carbohydrates amounts prior to meals for proper prandial dosing. In contrast, a fully closed loop system would automate all insulin delivery without the requirement of mealtime boluses or announcements.

Carbohydrate counting can be challenging, and patients' estimates are often inaccurate. Patients require a level of numeracy and literacy which is a potential barrier and is a burden for all patients. The elimination of carbohydrate counting in diabetes management would be of incredible value to PwD.

One significant challenge in developing a fully closed loop system is the need for information regarding timing and carbohydrate content of the meal to prevent significant post-prandial hyperglycemia following mealtime. Fully closed loop systems can be created using the same types of algorithms as hybrid systems—PIC, MPC, or fuzzy logic. Researchers have created algorithms to recognize unannounced meals and estimate carbohydrate intake based on glucose rate of change. Other solutions being looked at include integration of photos of food integrated into an MPC algorithm to help judge carbohydrate content of meals [11]. Some systems are currently looking to create "simple meal announcements" (SMA) to replace patients needing to input carbohydrate counts prior to meals. With SMA, the system will deliver partial boluses of insulin regardless of the carbohydrate content to be ingested prior to the meal and use automation to correct glucose as prandial response occurs. Unfortunately, current research has shown higher levels of post-prandial hyperglycemia compared to systems utilizing carbohydrate counting [10, 15].

Another significant challenge for fully closed loop system involves glucose control during exercise. Current systems allow users to set their pump to an exercise or activity mode which changes the algorithm target for a specified period. To be effective in preventing exercise-induced hypoglycemia, patients set these occurrences at least an hour in advance of the exercise. Biometric data such as heart rate, energy expenditure, and skin temperature have been used in trials of fully closed loop systems to recognize the type and intensity of exercise without any user manual input [11].

While recently approved faster acting insulin analogs including Fiasp and Lyumjev have faster actions profiles compared to Novolog and Humalog, research has only shown small benefits over standard insulin analogs when used in closed loop systems [7, 27].

Currently, the only commercially available fully closed loop systems are the STG-22 and STG-55 which are only available in Japan. Unlike the available HCL systems, these are bedside devices that use intravenous access for glucose sensing and insulin delivery and are limited to the perioperative setting for a maximum of a 3-day period [28].

References

1. Boughton C, Hovorka R. New closed-loop insulin systems. Diabetologia. 2021;64:1007–15.
2. Cinar A. Automated insulin delivery algorithms. From research to practice. Spectrum Diabetes J. 2019;32:209–14.
3. Moon S, Jung I, Park C. Current advances of artificial pancreas systems: a comprehensive review of the clinical evidence. Diabetes Metab J. 2021;6:813–39.
4. Templer S. Closed-loop insulin delivery systems: past, present, and future directions. Front Endocrinol. 2022;13:919942. https://doi.org/10.3389/fendo.2022.919942.
5. Hu R, Li C. An improved PID algorithm based on insulin-on-board estimate for blood glucose control with type 1 diabetes. Comput Math Methods Med. 2015;2015:1. https://doi.org/10.1155/2015/281589.
6. Thomas A, Heinemann L. Algorithms for automated insulin delivery: an overview. J Diabetes Sci Technol. 2022;16:1228–38.
7. Bode B, Carlson A, Liu R. 233-OR: Ultra-rapid Lispro (URLi) demonstrates similar time-in-target range to Humalog with the Medtronic minimed 670g hybrid closed-loop systems. Diabetes. 2020;69:233-OR.
8. Brown S, Raghinaru D, Emory E, et al. First look at control-IQ: a new-generation automated insulin delivery system. Diabetes Care. 2018;41:2634–6.
9. Forlenza G, Buckingham B, Brown S, et al. First outpatient evaluation of a tubeless automated insulin delivery system with customizable glucose targets in children and adults with type 1 diabetes. Diabetes Technol. 2021;23:410–24.
10. Haidar A, Farid D, St-Yves A, et al. Post-breakfast closed-loop glucose control is improved when accompanied with carbohydrate-matching bolus compared to weight-dependent bolus. Diabetes Metab. 2014;40:211–4.
11. Forlenza G, Breton M, Kovatchev B. Candidate selection for hybrid closed loop systems. Diabetes Technol Ther. 2021;23:760–2.
12. Messer L, Forlenza G, Sherr J, et al. Optimizing hybrid closed-loop therapy in adolescents and emerging adults using the MiniMed 670g system. Diabetes Care. 2018;41:789–96.
13. Messer L, Berget C, Forlenza G. A clinical guide to advanced diabetes devices and closed-loop systems using the CARES paradigm. Diabetes Technol Therap. 2019;21:462–9.
14. Lawton J, Blackburn M, Allen J. Improving management of type-1 diabetes in the UK: the dose adjustment for normal eating (DAFNE) program as a research testbed. National Institute for Health Research; 2014. https://doi.org/10.3310/pgfar02050.

15. Kropff J, Del Favero S, Place J. 2-Month evening ad night closed loop glucose control in patients with type 1 diabetes under free living conditions a randomized cross over trial. Lancet Diabetes Endocrinol. 2016;3:939–47.
16. Forlenza G, Carlson A, Galindo R, et al. Real-world evidence supporting tandem control-IQ hybrid closed-loop success in the medicare and medicaid type 1 and type 2 diabetes populations. Diabetes Technol Ther. 2022;11:814–23.
17. Bergenstal R, Garg S, Weinzimer S. Safety of a hybrid closed loop insulin delivery system in patients with type-1 diabetes. JAMA. 2016;316:1407–8.
18. Lunati M, Morpurgo P, Rossi A, et al. Hybrid close-loop systems versus predictive low-glucose suspend and sensor-augmented pump therapy in patients with type 1 diabetes: a single-center cohort study. Front Endocrinol. 2022;14:816599. https://doi.org/10.3389/fending.2022.816599.
19. Lunati M, Morpurgo P, Rossi A, et al. Hybrid close-loop systems versus predictive low-glucose suspend and sensor-augmented pump therapy in patients with type 1 diabetes: a single-center cohort study. Front Endocrinol. 2022; https://doi.org/10.3389/fendo.2022.816599.
20. Abraham M, Bock M, Smith G. Effect of a hybrid closed-loop system on glycemic and psychosocial outcomes in children and adolescents with type-1 diabetes. JAMA Pediatr. 2021;175:1227–35.
21. Wong E, Kroon L. Ultra rapid-acting insulin: how fast is really needed? Clin Diabetes. 2021;39(4):415. https://doi.org/10.2337/cd20-0119.
22. Burnside M, Lewis D, Crocket H, et al. Open-source automated insulin delivery in type 1 diabetes. N Engl J Med. 2022;387:869–81.
23. Berget C, Sherr J, DeSalvo D, et al. Clinical implementation of the Omnipod 5 automated insulin delivery system: key considerations for training and onboarding people with diabetes. Clin Diabetes. 2022;1:168–84.
24. Zeng B, Jia H, Gao L, Yang Q, Yu K, Sun F. Dual-hormone artificial pancreas for glucose control in type 1 diabetes: a meta-analysis. Diabetes Obes Metab. 2022;24:1967–75.
25. Peters T, Haidar A. Dual-hormone artificial pancreas: benefits and limitations compared with single-hormone systems. Diabetes Med. 2018;35:450–9.
26. Wilson L, Jacobs P, Ramsey K, et al. Dual-hormone closed loop system using a liquid stable glucagon formulation versus insulin-only closed loop system compared with a predictive low glucose suspend system: an open-label, outpatient, single center, crossover, randomized controlled trial. Diabetes Care. 2020;43:2721–9.
27. Boughton C, Hartnell S, Thabit H. Hybrid closed-loop glucose control with faster insulin aspart compared with standard insulin aspart in adults with type 1 diabetes: a double-blind, multicenter, multinational, randomized, crossover study. Diabetes Obes Metab. 2021;23:1389–96.
28. Namikawa T, Munekage M, Yatabe T, et al. Current status and issues of the artificial pancreas: abridged English translation of a special issue in Japanese. J Artif Organs. 2018;21:132–7.

Chapter 7
Diabetes Technology in the Geriatric Population

Michele Pisano, Nissa Mazzola, and Ngan M. Nguyen

Older adults are often defined as people aged 65 years and older [1]. According to the U.S. Census Bureau, more than 56 million older adults live in the United States, accounting for about 16.9% of the nation's population. By 2030, when the last of the baby boomer generation ages into older adulthood, it is projected that there will be more than 73.1 million older adults. The total number of adults ages 65 and older is projected to rise to an estimated 85.7 million by 2050—roughly 22% of the overall US population [2]. Almost a quarter of the US population will be age 65 or older by 2060 [3].

The major health problems facing the older adult population are also changing. The baby boomer generation has higher prevalence of obesity and chronic conditions, such as diabetes, than previous generations [2]. The Centers for Disease Control and Prevention (CDC) has recently released the 2022 National Diabetes Statistics Report. This report estimates that more than 130 million adults are living with diabetes or prediabetes in the United States [4]. Over one-quarter of people

M. Pisano (✉)
College of Pharmacy and Health Sciences, St. John's University, Queens, NY, USA

Northwell Health Division of Geriatrics, New Hyde Park, NY, USA
e-mail: pisanom@stjohns.edu; mpisano2@northwell.edu

N. Mazzola
College of Pharmacy and Health Sciences, St. John's University, Queens, NY, USA

Division of General Internal Medicine, Northwell Health,
Great Neck, NY, USA
e-mail: mazzolan@stjohns.edu; nmazzola@northwell.edu

N. M. Nguyen
Northwell Health Center for Liver Diseases and Transplantation,
Manhasset, NY, USA
e-mail: NNguyen4@northwell.edu

S. Fishman (ed.), *Advances in Diabetes Technology*, Contemporary Endocrinology, https://doi.org/10.1007/978-3-031-75352-7_7

over the age of 65 have diabetes, according to the CDC, and this number is expected to rise as the population continues to age.

Older adults with diabetes have a higher prevalence of comorbid conditions, such as hypertension, coronary heart disease, and stroke compared to those without diabetes. They also have a higher rate of functional disability, accelerated muscle loss, cognitive decline, and premature death [5].

Physiological Changes

Age is an important factor that can affect diabetes treatment. As people age, various physiological and metabolic changes occur, which can impact the management of diabetes. They tend to lose muscle mass and gain fat, which can also affect insulin sensitivity. This can also impact the efficacy of certain medications.

The most common age-related physiological change that can affect medication is a decline in renal function. Decreased renal function can impact the metabolism and elimination of some diabetes medications. This can result in an increased risk of medication toxicity, causing hypoglycemia and putting the patient at risk for falls. Adjustment to medication doses or the use of alternative medications may be required [5].

Other age-related changes such as decreased mobility, decreased physical activity, and changes in diet can also impact the management of diabetes. These changes may require adjustments to medication doses, insulin regimens, or other aspects of diabetes management [5].

Cognitive Decline

People with type 2 diabetes have a higher risk of cognitive decline and dementia compared to those without diabetes. Up to half of all older adults with DM also have cognitive impairment [5, 6]. Compared to patients with normal glucose control, people with diabetes have higher incidences of dementia. Uncontrolled diabetes and a longer duration of diabetes directly correlate to worsening cognitive function [7–9]. Systematic reviews and meta-analyses, with over two million participants, estimate that rates of all cause dementia, Alzheimer's disease [10], and vascular dementia [11] are higher for people with diabetes compared to those without. A large recent cohort study from Canada indicates that dementia risk is already increased in those with newly diagnosed diabetes [12]. Moreover, elevated glucose levels in individuals without diabetes have also been linked to increased dementia risk [13]. The Standards of Care in Diabetes 2023 recommends screening for early detection of mild cognitive impairment or dementia at initial visit, annually, and as appropriate in older adults [5].

Poor glucose control and complications related to diabetes, such as hypoglycemia and hyperglycemia, have been linked to an increased risk of cognitive decline. Vascular changes that occur in individuals with diabetes, such as damage to blood vessels and restricted blood flow to the brain, can also contribute to the decline. Vascular risk factors, in particular hypertension and dyslipidemia, may be associated with cognitive decline among people with T2DM although studies remain inconsistent [14]. Patients with poor glucose control and then manifestations of both microvascular (e.g., diabetic retinopathy) and macrovascular complications (e.g., myocardial infarction, stroke) are more likely to have worse cognitive function and are at increased dementia risk [14]. Insulin resistance, inflammation, and depression have also been identified as potential risk factors for cognitive dysfunction in people with diabetes [14–16].

Cognitive decline can make it more difficult for individuals to manage their diabetes, remember to take medications, and adhere to a healthy diet and exercise regimen. This can result in poor glucose control and an increased risk of complications. Older individuals with cognitive decline may have difficulty remembering the types and doses of medications they are taking for their diabetes. This can increase the risk of medication errors, such as taking the wrong medication or skipping doses.

Cognitive decline can also impact an individual's ability to make informed decisions about their diabetes treatment and management as well as their ability to recognize and respond to symptoms of hypoglycemia. This may result in poor adherence to treatment recommendations and an increased risk of complications.

To address the impact of cognitive decline on diabetes management, it is important for older individuals with diabetes to have support from family members, friends, or healthcare providers. Regular cognitive assessments, as well as strategies to support self-management, such as setting reminders and using technology, can also be helpful.

Hypoglycemia

Emergency department (ED) visits for severe hypoglycemia are now more common than those for hyperglycemic crisis and are associated with significant increase in healthcare costs [17]. This has caused diabetes care to shift its focus towards the prevention of adverse drug events (ADEs) associated with diabetes treatment due to the burden of severe hypoglycemia. In clinical practice, severe hypoglycemia is an episode that requires the support of a caregiver to increase blood glucose, usually by administration of glucagon or contacting a medical professional.

Hypoglycemia is a common risk in the older adult population, especially in those with diabetes and underlying medical conditions. Hypoglycemia in older adults is often underrecognized due to the prevalence of neurological rather than autonomic symptoms, presenting as dizziness or visual disturbances [18]. The risk is higher in older adults due to a variety of factors including decreased production of glucose by the liver, changes in insulin sensitivity necessitating insulin therapy and the effects of certain medications due to progressive renal insufficiency [19]. Lee et al. looked at 1206 study participants from the Atherosclerosis Risk in Communities (ARIC) study with diagnosed diabetes. Severe hypoglycemia was identified through 2013 by IC9-9 codes for hospitalizations, emergency room visits and ambulance use. During a period of 15 years, 185 severe hypoglycemic events were identified. Risk factors were age, diabetes medications (insulin and oral medications), kidney damage, and cognitive decline [19]. Older adults who take insulin to manage their diabetes are at a higher risk of developing hypoglycemia. Certain medical conditions such as kidney disease, liver disease, or heart disease can increase the risk of hypoglycemia. Some medications, including sulfonylureas and meglitinides, can lower blood sugar levels and increase the risk of hypoglycemia.

As stated earlier, older adults have higher rates of cognitive impairment, leading to difficulty adhering to complex medication regimens, glucose monitoring and insulin dose adjustment, they are also more likely to skip meals or have a poor diet that does not provide adequate amounts of glucose, which can lead to hypoglycemia. Glycemic targets and pharmacological treatments may need to be adjusted to minimize hypoglycemic events. Episodes of hypoglycemia should be addressed with both patients and caregivers and screened for cognitive impairment and dementia [5].

It is important for elderly individuals and their caregivers to be aware of the signs and symptoms of hypoglycemia, which can include sweating, confusion, weakness, and shakiness, and to seek prompt medical treatment if they occur. It is common to have a decreased central nervous system response as we age, which can contribute to hypoglycemia unawareness. In one study that looked at hormonal responses to hypoglycemia, people with diabetes over 65 years of age compared to people aged 39–64. The older age-group maintained hormonal responses to hypoglycemia but demonstrated more hypoglycemia unawareness. Since some older adults may have had diabetes for a longer period, this longer duration may lead to a lack of hypoglycemia symptoms, contributing to hypoglycemia unawareness [20]. In addition, it is important for older adults to regularly monitor their blood sugar levels, follow a balanced diet, and closely monitor their medication regimen to reduce the risk of hypoglycemia.

Safety of Intensive Glucose Control

According to the Standards of Care in Diabetes 2023, otherwise healthy adults with few co-existing chronic illnesses and intact cognitive function should have lower glycemic goals (A1C < 7–7.5%), while those with multiple comorbid conditions, cognitive impairment, and functional dependence should have less strict goals (A1C < 8%). However, hyperglycemia leading to symptoms should always be avoided [5].

This recommendation is supported by results of multiple randomized controlled trials, such as the Action to Control Cardiovascular Risk in Diabetes (ACCORD) study and the Veterans Affairs Diabetes Trial (VADT), which demonstrated that multidrug regimens and strict glycemic goals (A1C < 6%) had a significantly higher rate of severe hypoglycemia compared to standard therapy [21, 22]. Result of the ACCORD trial also showed that compared to standard therapy, the use of intensive therapy for 3.5 years increased mortality and did not significantly reduce major cardiovascular events [21].

Polypharmacy

Polypharmacy is a common problem in older adults, particularly those with diabetes. As the population ages, a higher prevalence of multiple comorbid conditions must be managed concurrently. According to the Centers for Disease Control and Prevention (CDC), older adults are the largest consumers of prescription and non-prescription medications, and this number continues to rise [23]. Polypharmacy refers to the use of multiple medications to treat one or more medical conditions. In older adults with diabetes, it is not uncommon for them to be taking multiple medications to manage their diabetes and other comorbid medical conditions. Factors that contribute to polypharmacy in older adults with diabetes are multiple medical conditions, pharmacodynamic and pharmacokinetic age-related changes, and cognitive decline.

Although there is no agreed-on definition of polypharmacy, some will say five or more medications. An alternate definition for polypharmacy can be the use of more medications than are medically necessary. While multiple medications can be helpful in managing multiple medical conditions, they can also increase the risk of adverse reactions and drug interactions, which can lead to increased hospitalizations and decreased quality of life. Older adults are nearly seven times as likely as younger persons to have adverse drug events that require hospitalization [24].

To reduce the risk of adverse reactions and drug interactions in older adults with diabetes, it is important for them to work closely with their healthcare provider to develop an individualized plan for managing their medications. This may involve reviewing their current medications to determine if any can be discontinued, adjusting doses, or switching to alternative medications that are less likely to interact with each other.

Visual and Hearing Impairment

Both hearing and visual impairments can make it difficult to use diabetes technology, such as blood glucose meters, insulin pumps, and continuous glucose monitors.

Hearing impairment can make it difficult to hear alarms or alerts from diabetes technology devices, which are important for managing blood sugar levels. This can lead to missed or delayed treatment, which can have serious consequences for people with diabetes.

Visual impairment can make it difficult to read the screens and displays on diabetes technology devices, which can make it difficult to properly use these devices. People with visual impairment may also have difficulty locating the necessary buttons or features on the device, which can make it difficult to perform routine tasks such as checking blood sugar levels or adjusting insulin doses. People with visual impairment may have difficulty reading the labels on insulin bottles or pens, which can lead to errors in dosing. This can be especially problematic if there are multiple types of insulin being used, as they may have different dosing requirements.

To overcome these challenges, people with hearing or visual impairments may require specialized diabetes technology devices that have been designed to accommodate their specific needs. For example, some devices may have larger or tactile buttons, or may have audio or vibration alerts instead of visual alerts. Additionally, training and support may be necessary to help people with hearing or visual impairments properly use diabetes technology devices, as well as to help them develop alternative strategies for managing their diabetes, such as using a talking blood glucose meter or relying on a caregiver for assistance.

The Prodigy Voice by Prodigy Diabetes Care is the only glucometer with comprehensive speech output throughout every step of obtaining a blood glucose measurement. It provides speak test results in about 6 or 7 s and has a repeat button in case you miss something that is spoken. It will alert you if your reading is out of the normal healthy range and automatically work with their strips (no need to code the meter for each new bottle of strips). All of the strips work with capillary action, which pulls your blood sample into the strip, eliminating the need to place a large drop of blood onto the specific spot on the strip [25]. Medicare will cover these glucometers under Part B coverage with a diagnosis code for diabetes and low vision or blindness [26]. Increasing awareness and accessibility for totally audible glucometers can help improve the lives of those who have diabetes and vision impairment.

mHealth

Mobile health, or mHealth, is an emerging field that uses mobile devices, such as smartphones, tablets, or wearable devices to improve healthcare delivery and patient outcomes. The use of mHealth technology in the elderly population is of particular interest due to the growing aging population and the need for innovative solutions to improve their health and quality of life. The use of mHealth for diabetes management in the elderly has gained popularity in recent years due to its convenience, affordability, and potential for improved outcomes. mHealth can play a significant role in diabetes management for the elderly.

mHealth Apps

mHealth apps can help seniors better manage their diabetes by reminding them when to take their medications and tracking their medication adherence. These apps can also provide information about dosages and potential side effects. mHealth apps can help seniors track their food intake, including carbohydrates, and monitor their physical activity, which can help maintain a healthy weight.

mHealth apps can provide seniors with educational resources about diabetes management, including information about healthy eating, medication management, and glucose monitoring.

Telemedicine

Telemedicine refers to the use of technology to deliver medical care and diagnostic and health services remotely. It enables patients to receive diagnosis, treatment, and monitoring from healthcare professionals without the need for in-person visits. This can include conducting diagnostic tests, closely monitoring a patient after treatment, and referring patients to specialists.

Alternatively, telehealth is a broader term that encompasses a range of healthcare services and technologies that support remote patient monitoring, education, and consultation. It includes not only telemedicine but also other tools like wearable devices, mobile health apps, remote monitoring devices, and more. It often involves services provided by nurses, pharmacists, or social workers, for example, who help with patient health education, social support and medication adherence, and troubleshooting health issues for patients and their caregivers.

Telemedicine refers to the use of remote communication technologies, such as video conferencing and messaging, to provide healthcare services to patients. Telemedicine can be used to monitor blood glucose levels, provide remote consultations, and deliver diabetes education and self-management support.

Benefits of mHealth in Older Adults

One of the main benefits of mHealth in the elderly is the ability to monitor and manage chronic conditions. Chronic diseases, such as diabetes, hypertension, and heart disease, are common in the elderly and can have a significant impact on their health and well-being. mHealth technologies, such as mobile apps and wearable devices, can be used to monitor vital signs, track medication adherence, and provide personalized health coaching to help patients manage their conditions more effectively. mHealth technologies can be customized to meet the individual needs of elderly people with diabetes. For example, mobile apps can be tailored to track their medication, diet, and exercise routine, provide reminders for appointments and medication, and offer educational resources on diabetes management. This can help to decrease the risk of missed doses and medication errors. For example, a study conducted by Li et al. found that a mobile app-based intervention improved medication adherence and self-management of diabetes in elderly patients [27]. Several studies have investigated the effectiveness of mHealth technologies for diabetes management in the elderly population. A systematic review evaluated the impact of smartphone apps on glycemic control in adults with diabetes. The review included peer-reviewed articles examining the use of mobile phones for diabetes management. The outcomes assessed varied, however, most results showed improvement in self-efficacy, self-management behaviors, and hemoglobin A1c. This review found that mobile phones can be effective to help patients better manage their diabetes; however, studies with larger sample size and longer duration are warranted [28].

Another systematic review and meta-analysis analyzed the effectiveness of mHealth interventions, or self-management health information technology (SMHIT), on HbA1c levels in older adults with type 2 diabetes. The review included 52 randomized controlled trials involving over 6000 participants. The authors found that mHealth interventions led to a significant reduction in HbA1c levels compared to usual care or non-mHealth interventions [29]. This meta-analysis also showed that the effect of SMHIT was significantly greater when the technology was a web-based application that was easily accessible from the home without location restrictions [29].

Another study was done to test the efficacy of an mHealth intervention, (Integrational Mobile Technology Opportunities Program, IMTOP), for older adults with type 2 diabetes in rural Taiwan. Participants used a diabetes self-management app to track health behaviors. Patients reported self-care behaviors, T2DM symptoms, clinical outcomes, health resource utilization, and medical expenditure. These outcomes were measured at baseline and at 4 and 8 months. Improvements in self-care behaviors were reported at 4 months in diet, exercise, smoking, and blood glucose testing. Improvements in fasting blood glucose and cholesterol were also observed at 4 months. Patients also paid less in both endocrinology visits and medications. At 8 months, a statistically significant improvement in diet and smoking were maintained [30]. A meta- analysis of 34 studies concluded that mHealth interventions, including mobile, computer-based, e-mail and internet approaches, had positive effects on glycemic control, both clinically and statistically in older adults with diabetes [31]. All trials resulted in a reduction in HbA1c among which 62.5% were statistically significant. Out of all technology this study reviewed, mobile phone-based approaches were the most effective in improving glycemic control [31].

A pilot study of a mobile phone diabetes intervention for diabetes self-management in elderly patients also showed promising results in improving glycemic control and self-management behaviors. This pilot study recruited patients 65 years of age and older, with T2DM, cognitively intact, and on at least one anti-hyperglycemic medication from a community-based primary care physicians office.

Seven patients were enrolled in the study. This study found that older adults were able to use mobile phones and patient web portals to input blood glucose values and diabetes self-management information. They were motivated to input and monitor blood glucose levels, diet, medications, and exercise. Self-efficacy improved; however, it was not statistically significant. This can be due to the small sample size. Although these results are positive, larger studies for a longer duration should be conducted [32].

Another benefit of mHealth in the elderly is the ability to improve access to healthcare services. Elderly patients often face barriers to accessing healthcare services, such as mobility issues, transportation challenges, and limited access to healthcare facilities. mHealth technologies, such as telemedicine and remote patient monitoring, can help overcome these barriers by allowing patients to receive care from the comfort of their homes. For example, a study conducted by Clark et al. found that telemonitoring was effective in reducing blood pressure in elderly patients with hypertension [33]. For patients with diabetes, they can use mobile devices to monitor their blood sugar levels, track their medication, and communicate with healthcare providers remotely. This can be especially beneficial for those who live in rural areas or have limited mobility.

In addition to improving healthcare outcomes, mHealth technologies can also improve the quality of life of elderly patients. For example, mobile apps can be used to provide cognitive stimulation and social support to elderly patients, which can help prevent cognitive decline and reduce loneliness and depression. Studies have found that tablet-based interventions improved cognitive function and quality of life in elderly patients with mild cognitive impairment and may delay cognitive changes [34, 35].

Telemedicine enables seniors to consult with healthcare providers remotely; this is especially beneficial for seniors who have difficulty traveling to appointments. Telemedicine can enable healthcare providers to remotely monitor elderly people with diabetes, detect early warning signs of complications, and intervene before they become severe. This can be especially beneficial for those who have difficulty accessing healthcare services or need frequent monitoring. It can facilitate communication between elderly people with diabetes and healthcare providers, enabling them to discuss their concerns, ask questions, and receive support remotely. This can improve the quality of care and reduce the risk of hospitalization. A meta-analysis of 127 randomized controlled trials indicates that the risk of all-cause hospitalization decreased significantly for condition-related hospitalizations. Telehealth leads to reductions in mean all-cause and condition-related hospitalizations. For hospitalized patients, the mean stay for any cause could potentially be reduced; however, there is low quality evidence to support this [36].

In addition, a randomized controlled trial for diabetes and depression management found that the pharmacist-led telehealth intervention improved cardiovascular and depression medication adherence over a 6-month period as compared to nurse-led usual care [37]. Veterans with diabetes (A1C > 7.5%), diagnosed depression, and access to a landline phone were randomized to either pharmacist-led or nurse-led telehealth. The nurse-led group was considered usual care. In addition to usual care, the patients in the pharmacist-led group received an in-depth medication review. At the 6-month follow-up, there was improved medication adherence for all medications in the pharmacist-led group; however, there was no significant change in A1C or depression scores [37].

One meta-analysis reviewing 42 randomized control trials looked at the clinical effectiveness of telemedicine in diabetes mellitus. From these 42 randomized controlled trials, 6170 participants were included. 3128 were randomized to usual care groups and 3042 to telemedicine intervention groups. Eight intervention groups utilized teleconsultation, while 34 utilized telemonitoring. Patients with telemedicine interventions experienced a significant reduction in HbA1c with type 2 diabetes experiencing a greater reduction than type 1 diabetes. This study also showed that telemedicine programs that are longer in duration (>6 month) produce better results [38].

Telemedicine has also been shown to improve access to diabetes care in rural areas where access to diabetes specialists may be limited. A study of older adults with diabetes in rural areas found that telemedicine consultations with endocrinologists improved glycemic control and reduced the need for hospitalizations [39].

A systematic literature review of 30 research articles from 11 countries looked at the effectiveness of mHealth to manage type 2 diabetes self-care among older adults over 50 years old. When mHealth apps were paired with wearable sensors, patient satisfaction was the highest since they did not have to manually enter data. When mHealth short message service (SMS) was utilized as an intervention, patients noted that messages helped them improve self-care behaviors. mHealth SMS with telemedicine visits to offer coaching, produced the strongest results. This intervention showed an improvement in BMI, weight loss, exercise, diet, disease awareness, HA1c, and healthy behaviors [40].

Barriers to mHealth in Older Adults

Elderly people may face challenges in accessing and using mHealth technologies due to limited digital literacy, cognitive decline, and physical impairments. Therefore, it is essential to ensure that mHealth technologies are user-friendly, accessible, and inclusive.

The use of mHealth technologies for diabetes management requires the collection and storage of sensitive health information, resulting in safety concerns for patients. Therefore, it is crucial to ensure that these technologies comply with data protection laws and implement adequate security measures to prevent unauthorized access.

The cost of mHealth technologies can be a barrier to adoption, especially for elderly people with limited financial resources. It is essential to develop affordable and sustainable models for delivering mHealth services.

The accuracy and reliability of mHealth technologies can vary depending on the device and software used. It is important to ensure that these technologies are rigorously tested and validated before they are used in clinical practice.

mHealth has the potential to revolutionize healthcare delivery and improve outcomes for elderly patients. By providing personalized and remote care, mHealth technologies can help elderly patients better manage their chronic conditions, improve access to healthcare services, and enhance their quality of life. mHealth can help seniors with diabetes manage their condition more effectively by providing them with tools to monitor and manage their glucose levels, track their food and physical activity, and connect with healthcare providers remotely. However, further research is needed to fully understand the benefits and limitations of mHealth in the elderly population.

Continuous Glucose Monitors

Continuous glucose monitors (CGM) measure interstitial glucose, allowing for near real-time measurements of glucose levels [41]. Interstitial glucose readings correlate well with plasma glucose though values may lag behind if plasma levels are rapidly changing [42]. Despite this, CGM allows individuals to observe their glucose trends more readily and provide alerts when glucose levels are out of range. This enabling patients to make informed decisions regarding their diabetes management [41, 43]. Recent advancements in CGM technology further permit devices to communicate with insulin pumps via Bluetooth. Such improvements in CGM design, enhance device flexibility and promote a prospective approach to insulin delivery [5]. For a more comprehensive discussion on continuous glucose monitoring use in adults, please refer to Chap. 2 “Continuous Glucose Monitors”.

The benefits of CGM were initially seen in adults and youth with type 1 diabetes on insulin pump therapy and/or multiple daily injections [42]. Results from these studies demonstrated reductions in HbA1c level and/or episodes of hypoglycemia when participants demonstrated regular use of CGM. However, these early studies had limited representation of older adults even though the American Diabetes Association (ADA) describes that older adults with diabetes have a greater risk for hypoglycemia than younger adults [5, 41, 42]. Studies have shown that older adults with type 1 diabetes demonstrate a greater frequency of hypoglycemia unawareness compared to their younger counterparts [44]. Observational studies further suggest that approximately 50% of older adults with long-standing type 1 diabetes spend at least 90 min of their day with hypoglycemia and 25% of these patients spend as much as 150 min of their day with hypoglycemia [44]. The ability to reduce rates of hypoglycemia in this patient population can have significant clinical implications as repeated episodes of hypoglycemia further leads to unawareness and can lead to physical and cognitive dysfunction.

Literature on CGM Use in Older Adults

One of the earliest publications of CGM use in older adults was from a small retrospective review by Argento et al. [45] conducted in 38 adults aged 65 years or older with type 1 diabetes or type 2 diabetes. Compared to standard blood glucose monitoring (BGM), CGM use was associated with a sustained reduction in HbA1c (from a mean A1c 7.6% to 7.1%, $p < 0.0001$) and decreased rate of severe hypoglycemia (from 0.37 to 0.12 per year, $p = 0.0007$) [45]. In a small group of nine patients who did not continue CGM use, lack of insurance coverage was the most common barrier. Patients who continued to use CGM were more likely to have insurance coverage compared to those who were not [45].

Another small study by Volcansek et al. evaluated the use of CGM in a small population of 25 older adults (mean age 67.6 years) with well-controlled type 1 diabetes or type 2 diabetes receiving multiple daily injections [46]. A statistically significant improvement in time in range with CGM use (66.3% vs. 76.9%, $p < 0.001$) and reduction in glycemic variability was observed. Time in hypoglycemia was also reduced with CGM use (9.6% vs. 5.2% $p = 0.041$) [46]. It appears that even in patients with well-controlled diabetes, there is an added benefit of stabilizing glycemia with CGM use.

The Wireless Innovation for Seniors with Diabetes Mellitus (WISDM) trial randomized 203 adults over 60 years of age with type 1 diabetes to CGM or standard BGM [41]. After 6 months of follow-up, there was a small but statistically significant decrease in the median percentage of time with hypoglycemia in patients using CGM, compared to standard BGM [41, 42]. The median percentage of time with glucose levels less than 70 mg/dL decreased from 5.1% at baseline to 2.7% for the CGM group while the BGM group remained unchanged from baseline. Differences between groups corresponded to a treatment group difference of −1.9% ($p < 0.001$) and reduction in time spent in hypoglycemia by 27 min per day [41]. Such differences were noted as early as 4 weeks and were maintained through the completion of the trial. The reduction in time spent in hypoglycemia was consistent across the age range of 60–86 years, across baseline HbA1c range of 5.6% to 10.8%, among those with and without cognitive impairment, and across at all education levels. This treatment effect was greater in patients with higher baseline time in hypoglycemia [41]. The benefit of CGM in reducing hypoglycemia was observed during the day and overnight, as well as in patients using insulin pumps or multiple daily injections [41]. There were also significant differences observed for hyperglycemia and glycemic variability. Patients with CGM spent 2.1 h per day more in target range (70–180 mg/dL) compared to standard BGM [41]. Though the risk of severe hypoglycemia was significantly reduced with use of CGM, the majority of patients using CGM did not achieve the less than 1% target for time with hypoglycemia recommended for older adults by the ADA Standards of Care [41, 47]. Nevertheless, among adults aged 60 years or older with type 1 diabetes, CGM use resulted in a small but statistically significant improvement in hypoglycemia over 6 months without increasing hyperglycemia [41].

In an extension of the WISDM study, patients continued or transitioned to CGM use for an additional 6 months with less intensive follow-up [48]. The treatment effect in patients who continued CGM were sustained while patients who transitioned from BGM to CGM use, saw reductions in time in hypoglycemia and improvements in time in range despite fewer follow-up from study personnel [48]. By the end of the extension study, patients in the BGM-CGM cohort, median time less than 70 mg/dL decreased from 3.9% to 1.9% ($p < 0.001$). Mean time in range was improved in the BGM-CGM cohort from 56% to 60% by week 52 ($p = 0.006$). Significant reductions were also observed in glycemic variability and hyperglycemia metrics [48]. There was a small improvement in hypoglycemia fear and glucose monitoring satisfaction observed in the CGM-CGM cohort from baseline to 52 weeks [48]. Similar to what was observed in the randomized control trial phase, patients in the extension phase were not able to achieve the target of less than 1% time in hypoglycemia set by the ADA Standards of Care [47, 48]. The additional follow-up observation demonstrated that CGM can effectively reduce hypoglycemia in older adults with type 1 diabetes for a prolonged period of time [48].

Evidence for the use of CGM in older adults with type 2 diabetes was assessed in a subgroup analysis of the DIAMOND trial [44]. In this trial, 116 older adults aged 60 years and above with type 1 diabetes or type 2 diabetes using multiple daily insulin injections (MDIs) were randomized to either CGM or standard BGM. At 24 weeks, HbA1c reduction was greater in the CGM group versus standard BGM (−0.9 vs. −0.5, with adjusted difference in mean change of −0.4, $p < 0.001$) [44]. There was also observed significant between-group differences in mean glucose, glycemic variation, and the average time within range, and in hyperglycemia, but not with hypoglycemia. It is believed that the low baseline incidence of hypoglycemia affected the ability to detect a difference between groups [44]. Despite no between-group difference was seen, the minimal incidence of hypoglycemia with CGM use was noteworthy given the significant improvements in HbA1c and glycemic variability [44].

The MOBILE study was an 8-month trial comparing the use of CGM to standard BGM in adults with type 2 diabetes being treated with basal insulin. In a post hoc analysis of 42 adults aged 65 years or older, CGM use was associated with non-statistically significant reductions in HbA1c compared to standard BGM (mean difference in A1c was—0.65%, $p = 0.13$) [43]. CGM use resulted in favorable increases in time in range of 16% from baseline versus −5% in the BGM group (difference = 19%, $p = 0.01$) [43]. By the end of the trial, more older adults spent 70% of their day within range with CGM use than standard BGM [43]. Incidence of hyperglycemic events were also lower with CGM use [43]. These improvements in glycemic outcomes were comparable to observations in adults less than 65 years of age. Of note, the amount of time spent in hypoglycemia was low in both age groups with little difference between treatment groups [43].

The Older Adult Closed-Loop (ORACL) trial was a small clinical trial with 30 older adults with type 1 diabetes using a hybrid closed-loop insulin delivery strategy [49]. In this strategy, the insulin pump automatically adjusts insulin delivery based on feedback from the CGM. Hybrid closed-loop insulin delivery resulted in higher time in range compared to sensor-augmented pump, equating to an extra 90 min per day in target [49]. The time in hypoglycemia, time in hyperglycemia, and glucose variability was less with the closed-loop strategy. The greatest benefit of closed-loop insulin delivery was seen overnight improving time spent within, above, and below CGM target range [49].

Boughton et al. also evaluated the use of advanced insulin delivery technologies [50]. In a small clinical trial with 37 older adults with type 1 diabetes, the use of hybrid closed-loop insulin delivery resulted in higher time in target range than with sensor-augmented pump. The additional time in range equated to an additional 2 h per day [50]. The time spent in hyperglycemia was also significantly lower with closed-loop use but not for time in hypoglycemia [50], contrast to what was seen in the ORACL trial [49]. Nonetheless, hybrid closed-loop insulin delivery with CGM is safe and can lead to clinically significant improvements in glycemia control compared to sensor-augmented pump therapy, without increasing the risk for hypoglycemia [49, 50].

Benefits of CGM Use in Older Adults

Currently, the evidence base for older adults is primarily in type 1 diabetes, but evidence demonstrating the clinical benefits of CGM use in older patients with type 2 diabetes is growing [5]. Across multiple trials, CGM use was associated with reductions in HbA1c [43–45], reductions in glycemic variability [41, 44, 46, 48], improvements in time in range [41, 43, 44, 46, 48], reductions in time in hypoglycemia [41, 48], reductions in incidence of severe hypoglycemia [45, 46], and reductions in time in hyperglycemia [41, 43, 44, 48], compared to standard BGM. The ADA Standards of Care recognize the need for additional literature on the role of CGM in older adults with physical or cognitive limitations who require monitoring of blood glucose by a surrogate [5].

Patient-Reported Outcomes with CGM Use in Older Adults

Across the various trials, CGM use and adherence was high though researchers from the DIAMOND study noted initial concerns with older adults demonstrating 6-month sustained use of CGMs [44]. At the final visit, 97% of older adults used CGM for at least 6 days per week. Assessed using a 5-point Likert Scale, patient satisfaction was shown to be very high with CGM use in the DIAMOND study which likely contributed to the high frequency of use. The perceived benefits were high while perceived hassles were few per the CGM Satisfaction Survey questionnaire [44]. Usage was also noted to be high in the extension of the WISDM study where CGM use was observed up to 52 weeks [48].

The population in Volcansek et al. of older adults with well-controlled diabetes was also evaluated on their perception of CGM use [46]. Satisfaction was reported to be high with CGM measured via questionnaires. Advantages of CGM use was perceived to be very common, with 95% of patients expressing improved sense of security with CGM use, 68% reported improved quality of sleep, and 82% willing to continue with CGM use after the study ended [46].

Barriers to CGM Use in Older Adults

Lack of insurance coverage was the most common reason for discontinuation of CGM use identified by Argento et al. in their study [45]. Access has been one of the biggest hurdles facing older adults who receive prescription insurance through Medicare [51, 52]. Prior to 2017, Medicare did not cover CGM at all, requiring beneficiaries to pay out of pocket for CGM. Beginning in 2017, CGM coverage was provided to Medicare patients with diabetes, so long as they demonstrated use of an insulin pump or the need for at least three insulin injections per day, measured glucose levels by fingerstick four times per day, and required frequent insulin adjustments [51, 52]. Beneficiaries were also required to visit their healthcare providers in person every 6 months for continued coverage. Following COVID-19, Medicare further relaxed requirements by no longer requiring in-person visits and no longer enforcing the need to frequently perform fingerstick though other criteria still exist [51]. Most private insurances cover CGM and some state Medicaid provide comprehensive coverage for CGM though experiences may vary.

Though high rates of CGM use were reported in studies, CGM devices may be complex as they often involve multiple components with varying lengths of usage [52]. Operating a CGM requires the patient understand how best to use the device and may require patients to know how to set up mobile applications and Bluetooth or when to change transmitters which varies with devices [52]. These may be challenging in older adults with complex late-stage disease or those who are frailer or have dementia [52]. Physiologic changes related to aging may present as barriers such as declining dexterity, or visual and hearing impairments may limit a patient's abilities to manually use the device or hear alarms [52]. Further CGM devices produce a significant amount of data which may pose a burden of interpreting and addressing critical readings on patients [52]. The ADA Standards of Care recommend that technology be periodically assessed, as the burden of implementation may eventually outweigh the benefits, particularly in those with declining cognitive or functional status [5]. Despite the barriers, Prasad-Reddy et al. state that if adequately trained by healthcare professionals, older adults can wear and use CGM to a high degree as seen in studies [52].

Smart Insulin Pens and Pen Caps

Patients who inject multiple daily doses of insulin are required to recall the timing and amount of previous insulin doses [53]. For those unable to recall this information, it can lead to overlapping insulin boluses and puts patients at risk for hypoglycemia [53]. The impact of hypoglycemia on older adults have been previously reviewed. Smart insulin pens (SIPs) were designed to overcome this barrier. SIPs are reusable injector pens that come with prefilled cartridges instead of using vials or disposable pens. The first pen with memory function capabilities was marketed in 2007. More recent iterations can calculate insulin doses, track when doses are given, provide alerts, and generate reports [54, 55]. Bluetooth technology allows for the automatic and immediate transmission of data from the pen to a smartphone application [54]. Information on insulin administration is then readily accessible for the patient, caregivers, or healthcare providers to review. Smart pen caps are add-ons to regular insulin pens and enable similar functionality as SIPs [54]. For a more comprehensive discussion on smart pen use in adults, please refer to Chap. 3 "Smart Pens".

The American Diabetes Association (ADA) refers to SIPs as connected insulin pens [42]. In the 2023 Standards of Care, based on expert opinion, connected insulin pens can be helpful for diabetes management and may be used in people with diabetes requiring injectable therapy [42]. More specifically, based on expert opinion, the ADA states that for older adults with type 1 diabetes, connected pens can be used to reduce the risk of hypoglycemia [56]. Literature describing clinical experience using SIPs or pen caps specifically in older adults is limited.

Literature on SIPs and Pen Cap Use in Older Adults

Adolfsson et al. performed a one-arm observational study to assess the impact of an SIP on insulin management and glycemic control in Swedish adults with type 1 diabetes [57]. Though the percentage of older adults included in this study was not reported, the median age was 40.1 years (range 18–83 years), suggesting that older age was not an exclusion [57]. After an average observation period of 223 days, there was a significant absolute increase in the time in target range with SIP use, translating to an increase in 1.9 h per day or 8.5% more of the day in target range ($p < 0.001$ for both) [57]. The observed effects equate to a relative increase of time in range of about 21% of the mean baseline level. According to the Advanced Technologies and Treatment for Diabetes Congress consensus, an approximate increase of 5% in time in range is associated with clinically significant benefits. The increase in time in range of 8.5% reported in this study is expected to correspond to an improvement in A1c of 0.4–0.7% [57]. There was also a significant reduction in the time spent in hyperglycemia, equating to a reduction of 1.8 h per day ($p = 0.003$) or −6.2% of the day ($p = 0.021$) [57]. Time spent in level 2 hypoglycemia was also significantly reduced by 0.3 h ($p = 0.005$) or −1.5% of the day ($p = 0.004$). There was no significant change in level 1 hypoglycemia. Bolus insulin dose was significantly increased from baseline while there was no significant change from baseline in mean basal insulin dose [57]. Glucose variability decreased significantly, indicating that the increased time in target range was driven by more consistent and stable glucose levels throughout the day [57]. The number of meals with missed bolus doses was reduced with the SIP by 43% from baseline ($p = 0.002$) [57]. This means, more patients were using bolus insulin injections with their meals [57]. The observational nature of this study and the unreported representation of older adults may lead to hesitancy in generalizing the results to this population.

Using the same Swedish patient population described by Adolfsson et al., an analysis of the effects of SIPs on direct, indirect costs, mortality, diabetes-related complications, and quality of life was performed by Jendle et al. [58] Direct medical costs include pharmacy costs, costs associated with diabetes-related complications, and concomitant patient management costs, while indirect costs are a result of lost productivity. The analysis showed that the use of SIPs was associated with improvements in mean discounted life expectancy of 0.90 years per patient and mean discounted quality-adjusted life expectancy of 1.15 quality-adjusted life-years per patient [58]. Treatment with SIPs was also associated with a delayed onset of diabetes-related complications by an additional 2.9 years, compared to standard care [58]. Combining direct and indirect costs, the projected cost savings with SIPs were expected to be Swedish Krona 497,995 per patient, the equivalent of $58,014 USD in 2021, versus standard of care [58]. Similar limitations previously mentioned from this observational study apply to the interpretation of these results for older adults using SIPs.

In a recent real-world analysis of patients with type 1 or type 2 diabetes, a change in severe hypoglycemic events was measured after initiating SIPs to a pre-existing therapy regimen [59]. Patients of all ages were included in this study, including a subset of 166 older adults aged 65 years and above, with a mean duration of diabetes of 30 ± 6 years [59]. In the overall sample population, the mean number of sensor-detected severe hypoglycemic events per week declined by 13% following implementation of SIPs, from 0.67 in the pre-SIP period to 0.58 in the post-SIP period ($p = 0.008$). Particularly for the subset of older patients, the mean number of sensor-detected severe hypoglycemic events per week declined by 31% after the implementation of SIPs, from 0.36 in the pre-SIP period to 0.25 in the post-SIP period ($p = 0.033$) [59]. The authors of this study estimated that the potential cost reduction for the entire population in this study per month associated with a reduction in severe hypoglycemic events for this population is $19,234–$98,915 USD, if 5–25% of these sensor-detected hypoglycemia result in a clinically significant event [59]. Cost savings are predicted to be roughly $12–$59 per SIP user per month, or $110–$551 per SIP user per year. Cost reductions considered potential cost savings due to intervention rates and costs from severe hypoglycemia-related hospitalizations, emergency department visits, and ambulance transportation.

Benefits of SIPs and Pen Cap Use in Older Adults

Though literature on SIP and pen caps use in older adults is limited, benefits of using SIPs are likely to be similar to that of the general population [60]. SIPs can be used to assess adherence through real-time logging of administered doses. Data may be stored and then readily shared to caregivers or healthcare providers allowing for accurate interpretation and monitoring of insulin administration [55, 60]. Using SIP-reported data, clinicals may identify barriers to adherence such as missed doses or overlapping doses, allowing the potential for simplification of insulin regimens to prevent risk of hypoglycemia and treatment burden [60]. Reminders and alert features are helpful to ensure timely administration, as demonstrated by Adolfsson et al. wherein the number of missed bolus doses was reduced following SIP implementation [57, 60]. SIPs further support patients on insulin therapy with dose calculators providing clinical decision support and the ability to dose smaller units ensures accurate dosing [60]. They allow for clinical decision-making by helping to calculate each dose based on current blood sugar level, carbohydrate amounts, meal size, active insulin, and setting prescribed by providers. From a safety standpoint, in addition to preventing overlapping doses, SIPs may notify patients if their insulin has expired or exceed storage conditions thus prompting patients to replace their cartridges. Such warnings will prevent the administration of expired insulin therapy enhancing safety. Though the general literature is lacking, there are obvious scenarios where SIPs are likely to be beneficial. These benefits are likely to be particularly useful in certain patients including older patients and patients with conditions or disabilities that may hinder self-management [60].

There's some clinical evidence in older adults with diabetes to support the use of SIPs increasing time in target range, decreasing time in hyperglycemia, and hypoglycemia [57]. SIP use may prolong time to diabetes-related complications and increases in mean discounted life expectancy and quality-adjusted life expectancy [58]. Specifically for older adults, incidence of severe hypoglycemic events was reduced following SIP use [59]. Though the current body of literature is in SIPs, pen caps have similar functionality.

Barriers to SIPs and Pen Cap Use in Older Adults

Overall usage of SIPs and pen caps is impeded by low provider and care team awareness of the utility of SIPs and lack of training [61]. In a mixed-method study by Ospelt et al., low provider awareness often led to the exclusion of SIPs and pen caps when clinicians discussed diabetes technology with patients. Sixty-three percent of clinics reported provider preferences or limited training as a significant barrier to using SIPs at their practices [61]. Low provider awareness may drive prescribing comfort and patterns [61]. Twenty-seven percent of clinics stated that a provider's comfort level in prescribing SIPs as a barrier [61]. Clinics who have not embraced SIPs are unlikely to have structured processes in place to retrieve reports from smartphone applications and interpret SIP-generated information [60, 61]. Further, clinics highlight the disconnect between the prescribing process and patient retrieval of SIPs from the pharmacy [61]. Clinics have also cited that telemedicine and remote monitoring was a barrier. In those with baseline low prescribing comfort and a limited number of patients already prescribed SIPs, telemedicine was seen as a greater barrier [61].

Patient-related barriers include insurance coverage and cost, SIP education and training, and smartphone availability [61]. Insurance coverage for SIPs is not universal and may vary. There is conflicting information on Medicare coverage for SIPs, as most older adults with diabetes are likely to have Medicare [60]. Out-of-pocket costs or copay may be higher compared to regular insulin pens [60]. Knowledge of insurance coverage and navigating the benefits verification process was a significant concern for providers in Ospelt et al. [61] As SIPs rely on smartphone applications, this may be a barrier for clinics who serve low-income patients [61]. Some older adults may not be familiar with smartphones or have caregivers who can use smartphones. As smartphone navigation and SIP pen use may require dexterity, usage may also be impeded by poor dexterity and moderate to severe cognitive dysfunction [60]. Maintenance of SIPs including changing cartridges, replacing SIP pens, and updating smartphone applications are additional considerations with the introduction of SIPs [60].

Insulin Delivery Systems

Insulin Pumps

Continuous subcutaneous insulin infusion (CSII), also known as insulin pump therapy is a notable advancement in diabetes technology. CSII offers an alternative for patients who require basal and bolus insulin to manage their diabetes. Doses are delivered through a flexible plastic tube called a catheter. For more information on insulin pumps, see Chap. 20. CSII has been increasingly used among the elderly population as an alternative to traditional insulin injections. However, there are both benefits and challenges to using insulin pumps in this population.

Benefit of Insulin Pumps in Older Adults

Improved Clinical Outcomes

One of the benefits of pump technology is improved glucose control. Considering the risk of hypoglycemia in the elderly population is higher, there is often concern for insulin intensification. One of the primary benefits of insulin pump therapy is improved glucose control. Insulin pumps can deliver precise and continuous doses of insulin, helping to regulate glucose levels and prevent high or low blood sugar. This can result in better overall glucose control and improved quality of life for older individuals with diabetes. Much of the data available for insulin pumps are pertaining to younger patients. Recently, two small studies in older adults have been published. The Older Adult Closed-Loop (ORACL) trial was an open-label randomized crossover trial in 30 older adults (mean age 67 years) with type 1 diabetes for an average of 38 years. This study compared closed loop to sensor-augmented pump therapy. The primary outcome, time in range (TIR) measured by CGM, was significantly higher in the closed-loop group (75.2% [SD 6.3]) than in the sensor-augmented pump group (69.0% [9.1]; [95% CI 4.4–8.0]; $p < 0.0001$), a difference that amounted to 90 min/day. The authors concluded that a hybrid closed-loop insulin delivery strategy was associated with significant improvements in time in range compared with sensor-augmented pump therapy [49]. Moreover, they found a decrease in hypoglycemia with the hybrid closed-loop strategy that while small, was significant. Another open-label, crossover design clinical trial in 37 older adults (≥60 years) compared a hybrid closed-loop advanced insulin delivery system to sensor-augmented pump therapy [50]. The proportion of time with glucose in target range was significantly higher in the closed-loop group compared to the sensor-augmented pump group (79.9% [SD 7.9] vs. 71.4% [13.2]), a result that was statistically significant. The improvement seen in the proportion of time in range was largely as a result of decreases in hyperglycemia. No differences in the rates of hypoglycemia were observed. Both studies inclusion criteria included older adults whose diabetes was relatively well managed (mean A1C ~ 7.4%) and had a similar study design. While the evidence is clear in the younger population, these trials offer the first evidence that insulin pumps can be used in an older population to improve glycemic outcomes.

A retrospective case note audit looking at 360 patients (mean age 67) on insulin pump therapy with at least 1 year of follow-up showed sustained A1C improvement up to 3 years. Patients with impaired awareness of hypoglycemia saw an improvement from 50% proportion reporting to 40.6% at follow-up ($p = 0.002$). In this group of patients, metabolic control was improved despite a higher prevalence of hypoglycemia unawareness [62]. While seemingly beneficial, use of these technologies should be regularly reassessed, as those with declining cognitive or functional status may not continue to confer similar benefit. However, 38% of the patients with type 2 diabetes in the Optimize Study had mild cognitive impairment [63] which could suggest continued benefit for use in that population.

Patient-Related Outcomes

Another advantage of insulin pump is the flexibility they provide in terms of meal times and physical activity. This can be especially important for the elderly, who may have a less predictable routine or have difficulty coordinating insulin injections with their daily activities. With an insulin pump, older individuals have the ability to adjust their insulin doses based on their needs, without having to worry about the inconvenience of traditional insulin injections. In a cross sectional survey of 30 older adults with type 1 diabetes (mean at 69), all participants reported that insulin pump therapy benefited their diabetes self-management pertaining to exercise. In particular, the benefit noted was related to flexibility of insulin dosing, no injections, convenience, and the options to adjust or interrupt basal insulin [64].

In addition to these benefits, insulin pump therapy can also improve quality of life for older individuals with diabetes. Among patients with type 1 diabetes, there is increased treatment satisfaction when using advanced technology such as insulin pump and glucose sensors, with increased feeling of safety [65]. Improved glucose control and increased flexibility can lead to better physical and mental health, increased energy levels, and improved overall well-being. While sample size was small, Barnard reported an improvement in quality of life scores at 6 months in comparison with baseline (92.4 vs. 86.9; $p = 0.01$), and participants with poorer glycemic control had significant improvements with prior dissatisfaction with treatment (34.3 vs. 31.6; $p = 0.01$) [66].

Benefit of Insulin Pumps in Older Adults

Cost-Related Barriers

Medicare Part B covers external durable insulin pumps and the insulin the pump uses under durable medical equipment if certain conditions are met. According to the CMS website, a patient may be able to get an insulin pump and supplies covered if the following conditions are met: The patient has completed a comprehensive diabetes education program, has been maintained on a regimen of multiple daily injections of insulin (i.e., at least three injections per day), with frequent self-adjustments of insulin dose for at least 6 months prior to initiation of the insulin pump, has documented frequency of glucose self-testing an average of at least four times per day during the 2 months prior to initiation of the insulin pump, and meets one or more of the following criteria while on the multiple daily injection regimen [67]:

1. Glycosylated hemoglobin level (HbAlc) > 7.0%
2. History of recurrent hypoglycemia
3. Wide fluctuations in blood glucose before mealtime
4. Dawn phenomenon with fasting blood sugars frequently exceeding 200 mg/dL
5. History of severe glycemic excursions

The other qualifying factor would be if the patient with type I diabetes has been on a pump prior to enrollment in Medicare and has documented frequency of glucose self-testing an average of at least four times per day during the month prior to Medicare enrollment. Patients with type I diabetes must be documented to have a C-peptide level of <0.5. For continued coverage of the insulin pump, the patient is required to have been seen and evaluated by the treating physician at least every

3 months. In addition, the pump must be ordered by and follow-up care of the patient must be managed by a physician who manages multiple patients with CSII and who works closely with a team including nurses, diabetic educators, and dietitians who are knowledgeable in the use of CSII. They include language on the website stating that subcutaneous insulin infusion pumps will continue to be denied as not medically necessary and reasonable for all patients with type II diabetes including insulin-requiring patients with type II diabetes [67].

Medicare patients who are prescribed insulin and using an insulin pump would use their Medicare Part B coverage for the cost of the insulin, whereas non-pump users will use their Medicare Part D Coverage. Effective January 1, 2023, out-of-pocket costs for insulin are capped at $35 per monthly prescription among Medicare Part D enrollees under the Inflation Reduction Act (IRA). A similar cap takes effect in Medicare Part B on July 1, 2023. An estimated 1.5 million Medicare beneficiaries who use insulin would have saved $734 million in Part D and $27 million in Part B if these caps had been in effect in 2020 [68]. In a national sample of privately insured patients with type 1 diabetes, mean (SD) annual out-of-pocket spending for diabetes-related supplies varied among patients who used insulin pumps only ($562 [$626]), continuous glucose monitors only ($472 [$625]), both ($1037 [$1039]), or neither ($79 [$175]). This study did not analyze data for patients with Medicare, so it is difficult to know whether Medicare patients would have more or less out-of-pocket expenses per year.

As you can see, one of the main challenges of insulin pump therapy is the cost. Even with Medicare coverage, the out-of-pocket costs may be burdensome as the patient is responsible for 20% of the Medicare approved amount after the yearly deductible. In a survey of 241 older adults with type 1 diabetes on Medicare, over 50% reported issues with access to supplies due to a delay in the release of supplies, paperwork issues, and difficulty seeing a provider every 90 days [45]. This also resulted in ill-advised behaviors like leaving the infusion site in for longer than 3 days and reusing pump supplies. As a result, erratic glucose levels and pain at the injection site were reported. These behaviors can contribute to injections, hospitalizations, and poor outcomes for the patient. These cost concerns can be a significant barrier for older individuals, especially those who are on a fixed income. Additionally, the cost of insulin pump therapy persists with continued use, as supplies such as insulin reservoirs, infusion sets, and batteries need to be replaced regularly.

Patient-Related Barriers

Insulin pumps can be complex and difficult to use, especially for older individuals who may have limited experience with technology. The process of setting up and using the pump can be challenging, and older individuals may need training and support in order to effectively use the pump. There are multiple buttons that need to be pressed for bolus dosing, and patients need to understand that all steps must be completed to ensure the dose is administered. Dexterity issues can pose a challenge although using insulin pens with reduced dexterity also poses challenges. In a study evaluating dexterity in insulin-treated patients of different age ranges, T2DM patients older than 70 years old had a higher prevalence of neuropathy. This contributed to consistently worse results with patients needing more time for the dexterity subtests as compared to the healthy controls [69]. It is important to assess a patient's ability to use the pump correctly before proceeding with training. While a published case report showed benefit in patients with type 1 diabetes and dementia in an assisted living facility, intensive training of staff, the patient and family was required to ensure safe use [70]. Insulin pumps rely on technology and can be subject to technical issues such as malfunctions, battery problems, or pump failures. These issues can be particularly concerning for older individuals who may have difficulty troubleshooting problems with the pump. Technical issues with the pump can result in disrupted insulin delivery and can lead to high or low blood sugar levels, which can be dangerous for older individuals with diabetes. With the initial evaluation, the physician and diabetes team should consider the following [71]:

1. Is the patient able to manage the technology involved with the pump?
2. Are there factors that would prohibit cartridge filling or infusion set insertions?
3. Is the patient (or care provider) able to troubleshoot problems that may come up with the pump?
4. What factors would result in CSII being discontinued for this patient?

Adults with diabetes, including older adults have shown hesitation about the inconvenience of wearing a device. In a survey of over 1500 participants enrolled in a diabetes clinical registry, were asked about their barriers towards device use and reasons for discontinuing a device. The most common reported barriers were related to wearing a device, such as the hassle of wearing a device all the time, and not liking having a diabetes device on their body as well as the way it looks on their body [72]. There is also concern that the device won't work and that they will need to devote more time each day managing diabetes [72]. With the evolution of smaller, sleeker, and more user-friendly insulin pumps, these barriers regarding wearability of the pump may be decreased, and be minimized further with increased education focusing on the potential benefits.

The time investment involved in pump initiation and use can also pose a challenge. Kamble et al. looked at time and costs associated with diabetes-related care between sensor-augmented pump therapy (SAPT) and MDI [73]. The analysis was performed based on patient-reported time collected over a 52-week period. Participants were asked to record the total time spent per week on diabetes management, considering different diabetes-related factors. The total time spent on the SAPT group was higher than time spent on MDI during and after pump initiation within the overall 52-week study. The reported weekly time estimates were as follows: SAPT 4.4 h and MDI 3.4 h (95% CI 0.4–1.7) [73]. The initiation period for the pump users (week 1–7) was 1.9 h more per week. However, all adults with T1D in the study reported that they spend considerable time on diabetes care.

Other Pump-Related Concerns

Diabetic ketoacidosis (DKA) is a life-threatening but preventable complication of diabetes, which is associated with an increased rate of hospital admissions. The commonly accepted criteria for DKA includes: hyperglycemia (blood glucose >250 mg/dL (≈13.9 mmol/L)); arterial pH <7.30 or serum bicarbonate <18 mEq/L and ketonemia (blood beta-hydroxybutyrate >3 mmol/L) or positive urine ketones [74]. Patients often experience nausea, vomiting, fast deep breathing and can have fruity smelling breath. They may also report fatigue and confusion. While the risk of diabetic ketoacidosis (DKA) is also a possibility with multiple daily injections (MDII), the risk is also significant with pump users. DKA in pump users is often a result of tubing or pump issues, such as kinking of the tubing, air bubbles, or dislodgement of the infusion set. While there are no studies specifically looking at the risk of DKA specific to an older population, a study was identified that aimed at identifying the cause of DKA comparing insulin pump users to MDII [75]. While not statistically significant, their results showed that the number of DKA episodes were more frequent in the group using MDII when compared with the group using CSII (52.2% vs. 25.0%, $p = 0.052$). The pump users also had more knowledge of DKA prevention. Omission of insulin bolus at the appropriate time, namely at mealtime, contributed to patients with T1DM being admitted with DKA. This was higher for the CSII group compared with patients with T1DM using MDII (90% vs. 30.4%, $p < 0.001$) [75]. Although the overall duration of hospital stay was similar, the use of an insulin pump was associated with a significantly longer MICU length of stay (LOS) compared with no insulin pump use (mean days 1.9 ± 0.62 vs. 1.3 ± 0.71, $p = 0.001$). Education surrounding DKA prevention and pump use is important for all patients to reduce rates of DKA in this population.

Skin integrity can be a challenge for longtime pump users or patients using multiple devices. Continuous use of the insulin pump can result in skin irritation or infection at the site of the pump. While much of the data on skin integrity is related to the pediatric population, this can be extrapolated to the elderly population as their skin is thinner and can be more likely to breakdown. One study showed that 90% of pediatric patients using an insulin pump longer than 4 months experienced dermatologic effects, such as pruritus, wound, and nonspecific eczema [76]. Older individuals who may have sensitive skin or a decreased ability to heal from injuries. Clinicians should assess skin integrity and sensitivity to adhesives and provide options to help overcome these barriers. Site selection and site rotation is also important to help minimize the risk of skin issues and lipohypertrophy. Skin irritation or infection can be painful and can make it difficult to continue using the insulin pump.

In conclusion, while insulin pump therapy can offer several benefits for older individuals with diabetes, there are also several challenges that should be considered. The cost of insulin pump therapy, the complexity of the pump, and the potential for technical issues, skin irritation are all important factors to consider when deciding whether insulin pump therapy is right for an older individual. It is important to carefully weigh the benefits and challenges of insulin pump therapy in order to make an informed decision.

Glucagon

Glucagon is a hormone produced by the pancreas that plays a crucial role in regulating blood glucose levels. It is used clinically to treat hypoglycemia, a condition where blood glucose levels fall below normal range. The American Diabetes Association recommends that glucagon be prescribed to all individuals at increased risk of level 2 or 3 hypoglycemia, so that it is available should it be needed. Level 2 hypoglycemia (defined as a blood glucose concentration <54 mg/dL [3.0 mmol/L]) is the cut off at which symptoms begin to occur and requires immediate action to resolve the hypoglycemic event [77]. Level 3 hypoglycemia is defined as a severe event that results in altered mental status and requires assistance from another person for recovery [77]. Family and caregivers should be trained on glucagon administration. Contraindications for glucagon use include patients with knows hypersensitivity or pheochromocytoma, which could results in secondary hypoglycemia related to catecholamine release after glucagon use. Nausea and vomiting are the most common side effects [78].

Traditional glucagon formulations have been available for several decades, but require reconstitution before use, which can be challenging, especially for individuals without medical training. In order to use correctly, glucagon and diluent must be first mixed together, then drawn into a syringe, then injected into the person experiencing severe hypoglycemia [78]. They can be administered as either an intramuscular or subcutaneous injection, with blood glucose concentrations expected to increase within 10 min. During the stress of severe hypoglycemia, these older glucagon kits can be overwhelming and confusing. This can be especially challenging for the elderly.

Until recently, there have been two traditional glucagon kits available in the United States, the Glucagon Emergency Kit (Eli Lilly) and the GlucaGen HypoKit (Novo Nordisk). Both were approved by the FDA in 1998 for severe hypoglycemia, with no age restriction. Recent advances in the development of new glucagon options have provided patients and healthcare providers with alternative options that offer several benefits over the traditional formulations. These glucagon options are designed to be easier to use and require little or no preparation. With more options available that are faster and easier to use, Lilly has discontinued Glucagon Emergency Kit (GEK) in all markets as of December 31, 2022 [79]. The generic GEK will still be available from Amphastar Pharmaceuticals.

Gvoke Xeris Pharmaceuticals

Xeris Pharmaceuticals has developed a ready-to-use, stable liquid formulation of glucagon, called the Gvoke Hypopen. It was approved in September of 2019 for the treatment of severe hypoglycemia in pediatric and adult patients [80]. This formulation is stable for up to 2 years at room temperature and does not require any reconstitution at the time of administration. This formulation is available as a prefilled autoinjector, similar to other rescue pen products like EpiPen, making it easier to use than traditional formulations. The injector is activated when pressed against the body, and there is no visible needle. There is a needle guard that automatically locks after use, an audible click when the medication is delivered, and a visual cue when the full dose has been delivered properly [81]. This formulation is intended to be injected subcutaneously into the lower abdomen, outer thigh, or upper arm. As with other glucagon formulations, emergency services should be contacted immediately after administration, and once the patient is responsive they should consume oral carbohydrates.

Traditional glucagon formulations have a rapid onset of action of about 10 min after injection [82]. Gvoke also works quickly to increase blood sugar levels, with effects typically occurring approximately 13 min after administration [83]. In clinical studies, Gvoke brought 99% of adults out of their very low blood sugar event [84] and was considered non-inferior to the traditional glucagon kit group. Gvoke demonstrated glucose Cmax, Tmax, and AUC compared to that of traditional glucagon kits [83].

Contraindications, precautions, warnings, and drug interactions comparable to traditional kits, with the exception of a skin rash that was reported in the package insert [84]. Necrolytic migratory erythema is a skin rash has been reported but more commonly seen in continuous glucagon infusions. It also resolved with glucagon discontinuation [84]. Gvoke is generally well-tolerated, and the most common side effects are similar to those of other glucagon products and include nausea and vomiting. Gvoke has been shown to be both safe and effective in clinical studies and is approved by the US Food and Drug Administration (FDA).

Baqsimi

Baqsimi (Eli Lilly) is a nasal glucagon formulation, which is used to treat severe hypoglycemia in people with diabetes. Baqsimi works quickly to increase blood sugar levels, with effects typically occurring within 10–20 min after administration. It comes in a single-use device that is pre-measured and does not require mixing or preparation. This makes it convenient to carry and use when needed. Baqsimi has been shown to be both safe and effective in clinical studies and is approved by US Food and Drug Administration (FDA). In a meta-analysis of ten studies in patients who are disoriented or unconscious, treatment with injectable or ready-to-use intranasal glucagon increased blood glucose within 15–30 min. In addition, intranasal glucagon was preferred by most caregivers and noncaregivers due to its ease of use [85]. Another study that looked at 75 adults with type 1 diabetes showed that intranasal glucagon was effective at treating hypoglycemia. The success criteria was defined as a rise in plasma glucose to ≥70 mg/dL or an increase of ≥20 mg/dL from the lowest glucose value within 30 min after receiving study glucagon, without receiving additional actions to increase the plasma glucose level. Success criteria was met by all but one intranasal visit, with a mean time to success of 16 min for intranasal and 13 min for intramuscular [86].

Contraindications, precautions, warnings, and drug interactions are the same as with traditional glucagon formulations. The most common adverse events include nausea, vomiting, headache, upper respiratory tract irritation, watery eyes, and itchy eyes, nose, and throats [87]. Considering this is a nasal spray, one may be concerned over the efficacy in the presence of nasal congestion. One study looked at the efficacy of the nasal glucagon formulation with nasal congestion as well as after recovery from cold, and there was no difference noted in blood glucagon or glucose concentrations. They also assessed whether use of a nasal decongestant would affect the efficacy of nasal glucagon, and no difference in blood glucose values was noted before and after a nasal decongestant was given [88].

Benefits and Barriers of New Formulations of Glucagon in Older Adults

Hypoglycemia poses a significant health risk and can often result in patients changing their behaviors to avoid hypoglycemia. In older adults, especially those with frequent hypoglycemia, it can result in cognitive and functional loss over time. Having easier options to offer to patients to overcome hypoglycemia can be of substantial benefit. Studies comparing the ease of use of both the nasal formulation and the autoinjector showed that caregivers were more likely to administer the autoinjector correctly compared to the traditional kit [89] and were more likely to feel comfortable using the nasal glucagon as it appeared easy to carry and did not require removal of clothing [90].

Cost, surprisingly, has not been a significant barrier for these new formulations. While wholesale costs for glucagon increased over the past decade, out-of-pocket costs have remained stable, as reported by researchers. In 2010, the average wholesale acquisition cost of glucagon hovered around $100 per kit and increased to just under $300 per kit by 2020, as reported in JAMA Network. Throughout this decade, the median out-of-pocket costs for traditional glucagon kits stayed at $0 for Medicare Advantage (MA) beneficiaries. But those in the top 75th percentile for out-of-pocket costs saw a price-tag of $25 in 2010, which later rose to $40 by 2020 [91]. The average wholesale cost unit is comparable to cost of Gvoke and Baqsmini, which average $368 and $336, respectively, for a single unit [92, 93]. Baqsimi, which was first FDA approved in July 2019, out-of-pocket costs were lower than unmixed glucagon for commercially insured patients. Median costs were $10.89 in

2019 and $15 in 2020. For Medicare Advantage beneficiaries, costs were $7.71 in 2019 and $10 in 2020 [91].

New glucagon options offer several benefits over traditional formulations, including ease of administration, stability, and rapid onset of action. However, the cost and availability of new glucagon options may present significant challenges that need to be addressed. Overall, the development of new glucagon options is a step in the right direction towards improving the management of hypoglycemia and enhancing the quality of life of patients with diabetes.

Conclusion

Diabetes is a chronic disease that affects people of all ages, but it is more prevalent in older adults. Managing diabetes in elderly patients can be challenging because of age-related complications, cognitive decline, and other comorbidities. Fortunately, diabetes devices have advanced significantly in recent years, providing seniors with various tools to manage their condition and improve their quality of life.

Continuous glucose monitoring (CGM) devices, which provide real-time glucose readings, are also gaining popularity among older adults. Insulin pens and pumps are other diabetes devices that can help seniors manage their condition. Insulin pens are convenient and easy to use, while insulin pumps offer greater flexibility and precise insulin delivery. However, seniors may need assistance in using these devices, particularly those with mobility or dexterity issues.

Additionally, telemedicine and mobile health (mHealth) apps have made it easier for seniors to track their diabetes management and communicate with healthcare providers remotely. Some apps even allow caregivers or family members to monitor their loved one's diabetes management from afar.

In conclusion, diabetes devices have significantly improved diabetes management in elderly patients. However, healthcare providers and caregivers must ensure that seniors receive adequate training and support to use these devices correctly and effectively.

References

1. Orimo H, Ito H, Suzuki T, et al. Reviewing the definition of "elderly". Geriatr Gerontol Int. 2006;6(3):149–58.
2. America's Health Rankings. Senior report. 2022. https://assets.americashealthrankings.org/app/uploads/2022-senior-report.pdf. Accessed 19 Jan 2023.
3. US Department of Health and Human Services. Healthy people 2023. https://health.gov/healthypeople/objectives-and-data/browse-objectives/older-adults. Accessed 1 Feb 2023.
4. Centers for Disease Control and Prevention. 2022 National diabetes statistics report. https://www.cdc.gov/diabetes/data/statistics-report/diagnosed-undiagnosed-diabetes.htm. Accessed 15 Feb 2023.

5. ElSayed NA, Aleppo G, Aroda VR, Bannuru RR, Brown FM, Bruemmer D, Collins BS, Hilliard ME, Isaacs D, Johnson EL, Kahan S, Khunti K, Leon J, Lyons SK, Perry ML, Prahalad P, Pratley RE, Jeffrie Seley J, Stanton RC, Gabbay RA, on behalf of the American Diabetes Association. 13. Older adults: standards of care in diabetes—2023. Diabetes Care. 2023;46(Suppl 1):S216–29.
6. Chaytor NS, Barbosa-Leiker C, Ryan CM, Germine LT, Hirsch IB, Weinstock RS. Clinically significant cognitive impairment in older adults with type 1 diabetes. J Diabetes Complicat. 2019;33(1):91–7.
7. Xu WL, von Strauss E, Qiu CX. Uncontrolled diabetes increases the risk of Alzheimer's disease: a population-based cohort study. Diabetologia. 2009;52:1031–9.
8. Yaffe K, Falvey C, Hamilton N, et al. Diabetes, glucose control, and 9-year cognitive decline among older adults without dementia. Arch Neurol. 2012;69:1170–5.
9. Rawlings AM, Sharrett AR, Schneider ALC, et al. Diabetes in midlife and cognitive change over 20 years: a cohort study. Ann Intern Med. 2014;161:785–93.
10. Zhang J, Chen C, Hua S, et al. An updated meta-analysis of cohort studies: diabetes and risk of Alzheimer's disease. Diabetes Res Clin Pract. 2017;124:41–7. https://doi.org/10.1016/j.diabres.2016.10.024. Epub 2016 Nov 9.
11. Gudala K, Bansal D, Schifano F, Bhansali A. Diabetes mellitus and risk of dementia: a meta-analysis of prospective observational studies. J Diabetes Investig. 2013;4:640–50. https://doi.org/10.1111/jdi.12087.
12. Haroon NN, et al. Risk of dementia in seniors with newly diagnosed diabetes: a population-based study. Diabetes Care. 2015;38:1868–75. https://doi.org/10.2337/dc15-0491.
13. Crane PK, et al. Glucose levels and risk of dementia. N Engl J Med. 2013;369:540–8.
14. Feinkohl I, Price JF, Strachan MW, Frier BM. The impact of diabetes on cognitive decline: potential vascular, metabolic, and psychosocial risk factors. Alzheimers Res Ther. 2015;7:46. https://doi.org/10.1186/s13195-015-0130-5.
15. Cooper C, Sommerlad A, Lyketsos CG, Livingston G. Modifiable predictors of dementia in mild cognitive impairment: a systematic review and meta-analysis. Am J Psychiatry. 2015;172:323–34. https://doi.org/10.1176/appi.ajp.2014.14070878.
16. Li JQ, et al. Risk factors for predicting progression from mild cognitive impairment to Alzheimer's disease: a systematic review and meta-analysis of cohort studies. J Neurol Neurosurg Psychiatry. 2016;87:476–84. https://doi.org/10.1136/jnnp-2014-310095.
17. Geller AI, Shehab N, Lovegrove MC, et al. National estimates of insulin-related hypoglycemia and errors leading to emergency department visits and hospitalizations. JAMA Intern Med. 2014;174(5):678–86. https://doi.org/10.1001/jamainternmed.2014.136.
18. Abdelhafiz A, Rodríguez-Mañas L, Morley J. Hypoglycemia in older people—a less well recognized risk factor for frailty. Aging Dis. 2015;6(2):156–67. https://doi.org/10.14336/AD.2014.0330.
19. Lee AK, Lee CJ, Huang ES, et al. Risk factors for severe hypoglycemia in black and white adults with diabetes: the Atherosclerosis Risk in Communities (ARIC) Study. Diabetes Care. 2017;40:1661–7.
20. Bremer JP, Jauch-Chara K, Hallschmid M. Hypoglycemia unawareness in older compared with middle-aged patients with type 2 diabetes. Diabetes Care. 2009;32(8):1513–7.
21. Gerstein HC, Miller ME, Byington RP, et al., Action to Control Cardiovascular Risk in Diabetes Study Group. Effects of intensive glucose lowering in type 2 diabetes. N Engl J Med. 2008;358:2545–59.
22. Duckworth W, Abraira C, Moritz T, et al., VADT Investigators. Glucose control and vascular complications in veterans with type 2 diabetes. N Engl J Med. 2009;360:129–39.
23. Centers for Disease Control and Prevention. The state of aging and health in America. 2004. https://www.cdc.gov/aging/pdf/state_of_aging_and_health_in_america_2004.pdf. Accessed 1 Feb 2023.
24. Budnitz DS, Pollock DA, Weidenbach KN. National surveillance of emergency department visits for outpatient adverse drug events. JAMA. 2006;296:1858–66.

25. Diabetes and visual impairment: an update on accessible blood glucose meters. AccessWorld®. 2012;13(2). Accessed 1 Mar 2023.
26. Centers for Medicare and Medicaid Services. Medicare coverage of diabetes supplies, services, & prevention programs. https://www.medicare.gov/Pubs/pdf/11022-LE-Medicare-Coverage-of-Diabetes.pdf. Accessed 1 Mar 2023.
27. Li J, Sun L, Wang Y, et al. A mobile-based intervention for glycemic control in patients with type 2 diabetes: retrospective, propensity score-matched cohort study. JMIR Mhealth Uhealth. 2020;8(3):e15390.
28. Holtz B, Lauckner C. Diabetes management via mobile phones: a systematic review. Telemed e-Health. 2012;8(3):175–84.
29. Tao D, Or CK. Effects of self-management health information technology on glycaemic control for patients with diabetes: a meta-analysis of randomized controlled trials. J Telemed Telecare. 2013;19(3):133–43.
30. Yu K, Wu S, Lee PJ, et al. Longitudinal effects of an intergenerational mHealth program for older type 2 diabetes patients in rural Taiwan. Diabetes Educ. 2020;46(2):206–16.
31. Yoshida Y, Boren SA, Soares J. Effect of health information technologies on glycemic control among patients with type 2 diabetes. Curr Diab Rep. 2018;18(12):130.
32. Quinn CC, Khokhar B, Weed K. Older adult self-efficacy study of mobile phone diabetes management. Diabetes Technol Ther. 2015;17(7):455–61.
33. Clark D, Woods J, Zhang Y, et al. Home blood pressure telemonitoring with remote hypertension management in a rural and low-income population. Hypertension. 2021;78(6):1927–9.
34. Li R, Geng J, Yang R, Ge Y, Hesketh T. Effectiveness of computerized cognitive training in delaying cognitive function decline in people with mild cognitive impairment: systematic review and meta-analysis. J Med Internet Res. 2022;24(10):e38624.
35. Vaportzis E, Martin M, Gow AJ. A tablet for healthy ageing: the effect of a tablet computer training intervention on cognitive abilities in older adults. Am J Geriatr Psychiatry. 2017;25(8):841–51. https://doi.org/10.1016/j.jagp.2016.1.
36. Peters GM, Kooij L, Lenferink A, et al. The effect of telehealth on hospital services use: systematic review and meta-analysis. J Med Internet Res. 2021;23(9):e25195.
37. Cohen LB, Taveira TH, Wu WC, et al. Pharmacist-led telehealth disease management program for patients with diabetes and depression. J Telemed Telecare. 2020;26(5):294–302.
38. Tchero H, Kangambega P, Briatte C, et al. Clinical effectiveness of telemedicine in diabetes mellitus: a meta-analysis of 42 randomized controlled trials. Telemed J E Health. 2019;25(7):569–83.
39. West SP, Lagua C, Trief PM, et al. Goal setting using telemedicine in rural underserved older adults with diabetes: experiences from the informatics for diabetes education and telemedicine project. Telemed J E Health. 2010;16(4):405–16.
40. Kruse CS, Mileski M, Heinemann K, et al. Analyzing the effectiveness of mHealth to manage diabetes mellitus among adults over 50: a systematic literature review. J Multidiscip Healthc. 2023;16:101–17.
41. Pratley RE, Kanapka LG, Rickels MR, et al. Effect of continuous glucose monitoring on hypoglycemia in older adults with type 1 diabetes: a randomized clinical trial. JAMA. 2020;323(23):2397–406.
42. ElSayed NA, Aleppo G, Aroda VR, et al. 7. Diabetes technology: standards of care in diabetes—2023. Diabetes Care. 2023;46(Suppl 1):S111–27.
43. Bao S, Bailey R, Calhoun P. Effectiveness of continuous glucose monitoring in older adults with type 2 diabetes treated with basal insulin. Diabetes Technol Ther. 2022;24(5):299–306.
44. Ruedy KJ, Parkin CG, Riddlesworth TD, et al., DIAMOND Study Group. Continuous glucose monitoring in older adults with type 1 and type 2 diabetes using multiple daily injections of insulin: results from the DIAMOND Trial. J Diabetes Sci Technol. 2017;11(6):1138–46.
45. Argento NB, Nakamura K. Personal real-time continuous glucose monitoring in patients 65 years and older. Endocr Pract. 2014;20:1297–302.

46. Volčanšek Š, Lunder M, Janež A. Acceptability of continuous glucose monitoring in elderly diabetes patients using multiple daily insulin injections. Diabetes Technol Ther. 2019;21(10):566–74.
47. ElSayed NA, Aleppo G, Aroda VR, et al. 6. Glycemic targets: standards of care in diabetes—2023. Diabetes Care. 2023;46(Suppl 1):S97–S110.
48. Miller KM, Kanapka LG, Rickels MR, et al. Benefit of continuous glucose monitoring in reducing hypoglycemia is sustained through 12 months of use among older adults with type 1 diabetes. Diabetes Technol Ther. 2022;24:424–34.
49. McAuley SA, Trawley S, Vogrin S, et al. Closed-loop insulin delivery versus sensor-augmented pump therapy in older adults with type 1 diabetes (ORACL): a randomized, crossover trial. Diabetes Care. 2022;45(2):381–90.
50. Boughton CK, Hartnell S, Thabit H, et al. Hybrid closed-loop glucose control compared with sensor augmented pump therapy in older adults with type 1 diabetes: an open-label multicentre, multinational, randomized, crossover study. Lancet Healthy Longev. 2022;3(3):e135–42.
51. DeCarlo K, Aleppo G. Perspectives on the barriers and benefits of diabetes technology in older adults with diabetes in the USA. US Endocrinol. 2021;17(1):1–8.
52. Prasad-Reddy L, Godina A, Chetty A. Use of continuous glucose monitoring in older adults: a review of benefits, challenges and future directions. touchREV Endocrinol. 2022;18(2):116–21.
53. Masierek M, Nabrdalik K, Janota O, et al. The review of insulin pens-past, present, and look to the future. Front Endocrinol (Lausanne). 2022;13:827484.
54. What is a smart insulin pen? American Diabetes Association. 2023. https://diabetes.org/tools-support/devices-technology/smart-insulin-pen. Accessed 14 Feb 2023.
55. Heinemann L, Schnell O, Gehr B, et al. Digital diabetes management: a literature review of smart insulin pens. J Diabetes Sci Technol. 2022;16(3):587–95.
56. ElSayed NA, Aleppo G, Aroda VR, et al. 13. Older adults: standards of care in diabetes—2023. Diabetes Care. 2023;46(Suppl 1):S216–29. https://doi.org/10.2337/dc23-S013.
57. Adolfsson P, Hartvig NV, Kaas A. Increased time in range and fewer missed bolus injections after introduction of a smart connected insulin pen. Diabetes Technol Ther. 2020;22(10):709–18.
58. Jendle J, Ericsson Å, Gundgaard J, et al. Smart insulin pens are associated with improved clinical outcomes at lower cost versus standard-of-care treatment of type 1 diabetes in Sweden: a cost-effectiveness analysis. Diabetes Ther. 2021;12(1):373–88.
59. Chien A, Thanasekaran S, Gaetano A, et al. Potential cost savings in the United States from a reduction in sensor-detected severe hypoglycemia among users of the InPen smart insulin pen system. J Manag Care Spec Pharm. 2023;29(3):285–92.
60. Sy SL, Munshi MM, Toschi E. Can smart pens help improve diabetes management? J Diabetes Sci Technol. 2022;16(3):628–34. https://doi.org/10.1177/1932296820965600.
61. Ospelt E, Noor N, Sanchez J, et al. Facilitators and barriers to smart insulin pen use: a mixed-method study of multidisciplinary stakeholders from diabetes teams in the United States. Clin Diabetes. 2022;41(1):56–67. https://doi.org/10.2337/cd22-0068.
62. Yeoh E, Beato-Vibora P, Rogers H, et al. Efficacy of insulin pump therapy in elderly patients. Diabetes Technol Ther. 2015;17(5):364–5. https://doi.org/10.1089/dia.2014.0360. Epub 2015 Feb 4.
63. Reznik Y, Cohen O, Aronson R, et al., OpT2mise Study Group. Insulin pump treatment compared with multiple daily injections for treatment of type 2 diabetes (OpT2mise): a randomised open-label controlled trial. Lancet. 2014;384(9950):1265–72. https://doi.org/10.1016/S0140-6736(14)61037-0. Epub 2014 Jul 2.
64. Chakrabarti CA, Alipoor MA, Segaran ST, et al. Exercise habits and glucose management among older adults with type 1 diabetes using insulin pumps. Acta Diabetol. 2022;59(6):865–8. https://doi.org/10.1007/s00592-022-01858-3. Epub 2022 Mar 1.
65. Waite M, Martin C, Franklin R, et al. Human factors and data logging processes with the use of advanced technology for adults with type 1 diabetes: systematic integrative review. JMIR Hum Factors. 2018;5(1):e11. https://doi.org/10.2196/humanfactors.9049.

66. Barnard KD, Skinner TC. Qualitative study into quality of life issues surrounding insulin pump use in Type 1 diabetes. Pract Diabetes Int. 2007;24(3):143–8.
67. CMS.gov. Insulin infusion pump decision summary. 1999. https://www.cms.gov/medicare-coverage-database/view/ncacal-decision-memo.aspx?proposed=N&NCAId=40&fromdb=true. Accessed 10 Mar 2023.
68. HHS.gov. Insulin affordability and the Inflation Reduction Act: Medicare beneficiary savings by state and demographics. https://aspe.hhs.gov/reports/insulin-affordability-ira-data-point#:~:text=Effective%20January%201%2C%202023%2C%20out,B%20on%20July%201%2C%202023. Accessed 10 Mar 2023.
69. Pfützner J, Hellhammer J, Musholt P, et al. Evaluation of dexterity in insulin-treated patients with type 1 and type 2 diabetes mellitus. J Diabetes Sci Technol. 2011;5(1):158–65. https://doi.org/10.1177/193229681100500122.
70. Allen N, Litchman M, May A. Using advanced diabetes technologies in patients with dementia in assisted living facilities: case studies. Cogent Med. 2017;4(1):1411632. https://doi.org/10.1080/2331205X.2017.1411632.
71. Stephens EA, Heffner J. Evaluating older patients with diabetes for insulin pump therapy. Diabetes Technol Ther. 2010;12(Suppl 1):S91–7. https://doi.org/10.1089/dia.2010.0024.
72. Tanenbaum ML, Hanes SJ, Miller KM. Diabetes device use in adults with type 1 diabetes: barriers to uptake and potential intervention targets. Diabetes Care. 2017;40(2):181–7. https://doi.org/10.2337/dc16-1536. Epub 2016 Nov 29.
73. Kamble S, Weinfurt KP, Schulman KA, et al. Patient time costs associated with sensor-augmented insulin pump therapy for type 1 diabetes: results from the STAR 3 randomized trial. Med Decis Mak. 2013;33(2):215–24. https://doi.org/10.1177/0272989X12464824. Epub 2012 Nov 5.
74. Kitabchi AE, Umpierrez GE, Miles JM, et al. Hyperglycemic crises in adult patients with diabetes. Diabetes Care. 2009;32(7):1335–43. https://doi.org/10.2337/dc09-9032.
75. Flores M, Amir M, Ahmed R, et al. Causes of diabetic ketoacidosis among adults with type 1 diabetes mellitus: insulin pump users and non-users. BMJ Open Diabetes Res Care. 2020;8(2):e001329. https://doi.org/10.1136/bmjdrc-2020-001329.
76. Berg AK, Olsen BS, Thyssen JP, et al. High frequencies of dermatological complications in children using insulin pumps or sensors. Pediatr Diabetes. 2018;19(4):733–40. https://doi.org/10.1111/pedi.12652. Epub 2018 Feb 26.
77. ElSayed NA, Aleppo G, Aroda VR, et al. 7. Glycemic targets: standards of care in Diabetes—2023. Diabetes Care. 2023;46(Suppl 1):S97–S110.
78. GlucaGen [Package Insert]. Plainsboro, NJ: Novo-Nordisk; 2018.
79. Sommi A. As glucagon options expand, Lily discontinues emergency kit. diaTribe Learn. 2022. https://diatribe.org/glucagon-options-expand-lilly-discontinues-emergency-kit Accessed 4 Mar 2023.
80. Beyond Type 1 Diabetes Editorial Team. Gvoke Hypopen now available. https://beyondtype1.org/gvoke-hypopen-available/. Accessed 10 Mar 2023.
81. Newswanger B, Ammons S, Phadnis N, et al. Development of a highly stable, nonaqueous glucagon formulation for delivery via infusion pump systems. J Diabetes Sci Technol. 2015;9(1):24–33. https://doi.org/10.1177/1932296814565131.
82. Hawkes CP, De Leon DD, Rickels MR. Novel preparations of glucagon for the prevention and treatment of hypoglycemia. Curr Diab Rep. 2019;19(10):97. https://doi.org/10.1007/s11892-019-1216-4.
83. Gvoke [Package Insert]. Chicago, IL: Xeris Pharmaceuticals; 2021.
84. Christiansen MP. A phase 3 comparison of a novel liquid glucagon autoinjector to glucagon emergency kit for the treatment of severe hypoglycemia. Presented at the 78th Scientific Sessions of the American Association. Orlando FL, 22–26 June 2018. 2018.
85. Singh-Franco D, Moreau C, Levin AD, et al. Efficacy and usability of intranasal glucagon for the management of hypoglycemia in patients with diabetes: a systematic review. Clin Ther. 2020;42(9):e177–208.

86. Rickels MR, Ruedy KJ, Foster NC, et al., T1D Exchange Intranasal Glucagon Investigators. Intranasal glucagon for treatment of insulin-induced hypoglycemia in adults with type 1 diabetes: a randomized crossover noninferiority study. Diabetes Care. 2016;39(2):264–70. https://doi.org/10.2337/dc15-1498. Epub 2015 Dec 17.
87. Baqsimi [Package Insert]. Indianapolis, IN: Eli Lily and Company; 2019.
88. Guzman CB, Dulude H, Piché C, et al. Effects of common cold and concomitant administration of nasal decongestant on the pharmacokinetics and pharmacodynamics of nasal glucagon in otherwise healthy participants: a randomized clinical trial. Diabetes Obes Metab. 2018;20(3):646–53. https://doi.org/10.1111/dom.13134. Epub 2017 Nov 19.
89. Valentine V, Newswanger B, Prestrelski S, et al. Human factors usability and validation studies of a glucagon autoinjector in a simulated severe hypoglycemia rescue situation. Diabetes Technol Ther. 2019;21(9):522–30. https://doi.org/10.1089/dia.2019.0148. Epub 2019 Jun 20.
90. Bajpai SK, Cambron-Mellott MJ, Peck E, et al. Perceptions about glucagon delivery devices for severe hypoglycemia: qualitative research with patients, caregivers, and acquaintances. Clin Ther. 2019;41(10):2073–2089.e6. https://doi.org/10.1016/j.clinthera.2019.08.006. Epub 2019 Sep 13.
91. Zupa M, et al. Trends in out-of-pocket cost of glucagon, 2010–2020. JAMA Netw Open. 2022;5:e2229428. https://doi.org/10.1001/jamanetworkopen.2022.29428.
92. Lexicomp. Pricing (US) Baqsimi. online.lexi.com. Accessed 2 Mar 2023.
93. Lexicomp. Pricing (US) Gvoke. online.lexi.com. Accessed 2 Mar 2023.

Chapter 8
Diabetes Do-It-Yourself (DIY) Technology

Tasfia Hoque

The development of technology to manage diabetes has advanced significantly over the past few years. These technologies aim to create effective and intuitive treatment alternatives for patients with diabetes beyond multiple daily insulin injections. Despite the advancements, patients with type 1 diabetes (T1D) still face numerous difficulties in effectively managing their blood sugar levels. The #WeAreNotWaiting movement which developed the DIY artificial pancreas systems (DIYAPS) grew from innovation-minded patients with T1D who are unsatisfied with the current standards of care [1]. In order to achieve less cumbersome glycemic control and improved quality of life, highly motivated and tech-savvy members of the diabetes community began creating their own "artificial pancreas" systems that integrate continuous glucose monitoring (CGM), insulin pumps, and smartphone technology. Patients with diabetes and their families and caregivers congregated online and in-person in 2013 under the hashtag #WeAreNotWaiting to share information about open-source hardware and software solutions [1]. Many improvements in diabetes care have emerged from this movement such as monitoring CGM data from a smartwatch, remotely tracking children's blood glucose levels, integration of louder low glucose warnings, and treatment suggestions based on CGM data analysis to achieve automated management of insulin. Eventually tech-savvy members and supporters of the T1D community began creating their own closed-loop systems for automatic insulin delivery or open-source artificial pancreas technology. Today, there are a number of do-it-yourself (DIY) diabetes technologies created by members of the diabetic community. These technologies are frequently developed utilizing open-source hardware and software and are produced outside of the conventional medical device industry [2].

T. Hoque (✉)
KPC Health, Hemet Global Medical Center, Hemet, CA, USA

S. Fishman (ed.), *Advances in Diabetes Technology*, Contemporary Endocrinology, https://doi.org/10.1007/978-3-031-75352-7_8

Origins of OpenAPS

The "Artificial Pancreas" and Open Artificial Pancreas System (OpenAPS) are innovations that arose out of the need for safer and more streamlined glucose monitoring and insulin administration. It consists of three basic parts: a continuous glucose monitor (CGM), an insulin pump, and a small computer that links the CGM and pump together and allows them to work in concert [3]. A "code" entered into the small computer allows it to recognize what normal blood sugar ranges are and algorithmically determine how much and when to administer insulin. The small computer is also able to predict changes in blood glucose levels and recommend doses in advance of administration based on the prior CGM and insulin dose data. The artificial pancreas and the code used to run it allow individuals with T1D to operate both devices in concert rather than separately. One of the earliest DIY developments was the development of an online portal that can store and react to CGM data. The initial impetus for this hack was a lack of volume control of built-in CGM alarms to alert patients with critically low glucose while sleeping. Sending CGM data to the cloud allowed for a connection to a louder alarm and avoidance of a life-threatening situation. Subsequently, a different developer created a way to link the cloud data to an insulin pump to remove the human factor of self-adjusting and administering insulin. This created a "closed loop." [1]

Availability to Public

The high volume alarm and the completion of the closed-loop system can be traced back to 2013–2016. Unfortunately, the OpenAPS had not undergone the rigorous FDA approval process for it to be manufactured and sold commercially in the United States. In 2013, the #wearenotwaiting movement was founded to express frustration with the long regulatory process of having these life-saving medical devices approved [3, 1]. A key part of this movement was to make the software needed to operate the artificial pancreas available to the public for free. Additionally, the design for the original computer that allowed the CGM and insulin pump to work together in a closed loop was made available to the public as well. The community that arose from this movement continued to develop more sophisticated software as well as more affordable versions of the computers to help others with T1D automate control of their blood sugar levels.

Despite the movement, it took 3 years for the FDA to approve its first artificial pancreas system (APS), the Medtronic Minimed 670G system, in 2016. Since then multiple other systems have received FDA approval, including a second generation of Medtronic's original APS. The FDA also approved the TidePool loop, an app that contains the algorithm to automate insulin dosing. Artificial pancreas systems remain an ongoing field of investigation and innovation for the public open-source communities and the medical device industry [3, 1].

Evolution of DIY Technology

Nightscout

One of the pioneers of the DIY technology movement is the father of a T1D patient, John Costick, a software programmer. Costick's original goal was to monitor his 4 year-old son's blood glucose in real time. The Nightscout project dates back to February 2013 when Costick, with the help of an engineer, Lane Desborough, was able to create code that could upload the CGM's data into a computing cloud via a smartphone every 5 min. John Costik sent data from the Dexcom G4 CGM to the cloud using a combination of open-source software and technologies. The receiver that comes with the Dexcom G4 collects and shows local glucose data. The intermediary device was an Android smartphone. The Android phone was connected to the Dexcom receiver via a USB On-The-Go connector. He collected glucose data from the Dexcom receiver using a customized Android app named xDrip. xDrip was an open-source app made to communicate data and interact with Dexcom CGMs. The glucose data was transmitted to a cloud-based database via the xDrip app. The glucose data stored in the cloud was retrieved and displayed on the Nightscout website. This allowed Costick to view his son's blood glucose values via phone or web in real time. At that time, there were no readily accessible mobile applications that were able to access the data in real time. After he was successful with this project, he tweeted about it via social media platform, Twitter which was seen by others who were also skilled in computer coding and they collectively began utilizing, modifying, and developing new code to produce innovative and specific mobile technology solutions. Costick then went on to create the Nightscout Website which included setup code and instructions on how to set up the system. They also made a Facebook group titled "CGM in the Cloud" which served as a community platform for users to ask and answer questions from one another [1].

OpenAPS

In December 2013, Dana Lewis and her husband, Scott Leibrand, took the first steps toward making OpenAPS when they were frustrated with the low sugar level alarm on Dana's CGM. They began by obtaining the Nightscout software from John Costik that allowed them to upload CGM data to the cloud which then would connect to a louder alarm. The couple went on to develop an algorithm that would help calculate the amount of insulin needed based on the blood sugar levels. The couple then worked with Ben West to reverse engineer the communication of certain insulin pumps which allowed the CGM and insulin pumps to "talk" with each other, this created a "closed loop" and OpenAPS was born. The data from the CGM could be used by the computer algorithm to predict impending blood glucose values and send insulin dosing commands to the pump to try to bring blood glucose levels into the optimal range [3, 1].

OpenAPS refers to "open source artificial pancreas." It was made free online to the public by the developers for individuals that wanted to have seamless management of their T1D. The computer Lewis and Leibrand used is commercially known as the Raspberry Pi, and another commonly used single board computer was the Intel Edison. The need for an additional device on hand, a single board computer and its battery, and a communication USB stick (to send commands to the insulin pump) were the main drawbacks of this first iteration of the artificial pancreas. T1D patients using OpenAPS would have to purchase a piece of equipment and then manage carrying it with already having to manage their insulin pump and CGM [3, 1].

LoopDocs

The natural progression of the DIY pancreas, eliminating the computer, came in the form of the Loop system created by Nate Racklyeft and Pete Schwamb. The Loop app, which runs on an iPhone, acts as the system's central processing unit, in lieu of the single board computer. The application houses the OpenAPS algorithm that analyzes CGM data and generates suggestions for administering insulin. The insulin pump used by the Loop system is normally a compatible pump that is connected to the Loop app via bluetooth. A small device that enables interaction between the pump, iPhone, and the CGM, called the Rileylink, is required to run the application. Therefore, without the user's involvement and need for a single board computer, the Loop app is able to administer insulin and make insulin dose changes. The drawbacks with this system, again lies with requiring an external component to allow communication between the devices which has to be with the person at all times. Furthermore, Rileylink only works with select insulin pumps. This may require users to switch and familiarize themselves with a new pump. Additionally, the application is not FDA approved and therefore not easily accessible via the app marketplace. Interested individuals must register with Apple as a "developer" and then be able to build the application on one's phone using instructions available online [1].

AAPS

Predictably, a DIY closed-loop system was created for Google Android smartphones, known as AndroidAPS (AAPS). It was unique in that it didn't need a Rileylink type intermediary to allow communication between the AndroidAPS app, an insulin pump, and a CGM. Based on CGM measurements, the app automates the supply of insulin. AndroidAPS has a vibrant user community and options for customization.

Tide Pool

Tide Pool is an application developed in 2020 to allow smartphones or desktop/laptop computers to act as the intermediary that runs the algorithms to monitor blood glucose and administer insulin for T1D patients. The app only recently received FDA approval (January 2023) and works with every brand of CGM and insulin pump available in the United States as well as many blood glucose meters. The ease of having the data on one application allows the patient to see both CGM and insulin pump data side by side, view data over various time intervals, and add notes or context about what may have been occurring during changes in glucose levels (exercise, stress, etc.). One of the more unique factors about applications that will work across multiple devices, such as Tide Pool, is data gathered from users. Users that allow anonymous sharing of their data can help guide research about managing T1D and provide more information for the application(s) to predict glucose levels and administer insulin.

The components needed to use Tidepool are commercially available insulin pumps, a continuous glucose monitor (CGM), and a RileyLink that connects the two. Since Tidepool Loop is a closed-loop system, it may automatically modify insulin dosage in response to current CGM data. Through the adjustment of insulin delivery rates, the system seeks to maintain blood glucose levels within a target range. To utilize Tidepool's services, users are able to create a free Tidepool account which becomes the storehouse for their diabetes data. Users are able to upload data onto their account either via the Tidepool Uploader (program on their computer) or Tidepool Mobile (app on their phone). The Tidepool Uploader is a computer program that works with a wide range of diabetes devices including Omnipod, Dexcom, T-slim, Medtronic, etc. The user can safely upload and store their data in their Tidepool account by downloading the free Tidepool Uploader tool, connecting the device to the computer and then uploading the data from these devices. Tidepool Mobile app that can be used by iPhone and Android users works with the Tidepool Data Platform. With the Tidepool Mobile app, users can annotate meals, enter carbohydrates to be consumed during meals, create favorite foods, or enter workouts they are about to complete. After entering this data they are also able to analyze the results and get insight to their blood glucose trends. Tidepool Loop uses an advanced algorithm to evaluate CGM data and determine the appropriate insulin dosage. To calculate how much insulin is needed, the system takes into account user input parameters, trends, and current glucose levels. Tidepool Loop is an open-source project, where the users and developers can see, alter, and make contributions to the program's code. Innovators and teamwork are encouraged in the diabetes community by this accessible approach.

Current State of DIY Technology

Factors Supporting DIY Technology

OpenAPS and its other iterations have a robust community of volunteers working toward making the lives of individuals living with T1D better. The codes and data to create and run the various applications and machines mentioned above are largely available for free. The community is also able to assist in procurement of devices such as the single board computers or the Rileylink which may be hard to find or too pricey for some.

Besides the accessibility and support of an online community, DIY technology is specifically designed to make quality of life better for T1D patients. The steps of manually monitoring blood glucose, to decide what insulin dose would be best suited for the given scenario, incorporating past responses to insulin doses and meals into insulin dosing, and monitoring overnight blood glucose levels can be burdensome, especially for the very young or very old. This all becomes streamlined with alerts and suggestions from a smartphone application continuously monitoring and running an algorithm for the patient.

Factors Against DIY Technology

Despite a robust community of volunteers working toward improving access to this innovative technology, the FDA's stringent regulatory process has limited accessibility in the United States. For example, the iPhone application for Loop is not FDA approved, thus requiring purchase as an "app developer" followed by searching the online community for the code and instructions to create and run the application and connect the CGM and insulin pumps needed. These steps may be cumbersome for individuals lacking familiarity and comfort with technology. Furthermore, many pumps that can be "hacked" by users are older, out-of-warranty pumps that can fail when linked to the various devices above, especially in the hands of a user that is not technically competent.

The lack of regulatory oversight on the devices and applications that are not formally approved puts healthcare providers in a difficult place as well. Even if there are clear benefits to the patient, a healthcare provider could potentially be subjected to legal recourse in the event the patient experiences an adverse event while using non-FDA approved therapies. The relative novelty of these devices and applications also makes reliable long-term data for safety and effectiveness lacking. This again places physicians and regulatory boards at a disadvantage when providing recommendations and counseling.

Research on DIY Technology

In Gawrecki et al.'s single center clinical trial, the safety and glycemic control of Hybrid Closed Loop (HCL) for T1D was investigated. The HCL used in the study was the Do-It-Yourself Artificial Pancreas System (DIY APS) running on the AndroidAPS application. The trial began with a 3-week run-in period (training participant on the use of the system) followed by a 12-week period in real-life conditions. During the study, *no* episodes of severe hypoglycemia or ketoacidosis occurred. The study also found that the average sensor glycemia and the standard deviation of glycemia significantly decreased when compared to baseline ($p = 0.002$ and $p = 0.006$, respectively). The time in range of 70–140 mg/dL and 70–180 mg/dL of glucose also significantly improved compared to baseline (both $p < 0.001$). HbA1c and serum fructosamine concentration both improved at the end of the study period with both showing statistically significant changes (both $p < 0.001$). Gawrecki et al. stated their study demonstrated using "DIY APS based on AndroidAPS in highly-selected, closely monitored patients with type 1 diabetes is safe." The study also showed that multiple parameters used to assess metabolic control of diabetes improved (time in range, average glycemia, and HbA1c). One of the main goals of the study was to show that, despite lacking approval from regulatory authorities and having multiple devices from different manufacturers, patients were able to learn how to combine and use the DIY APS effectively. Secondary endpoints of the study were also promising; this included following glycemic variability. The average HbA1c of patients entering the study was 6.8%, which decreased by a statistically significant 0.5%. This decrease was reached without an increased rate of hypoglycemia (<54 or <70 mg/dL) from baseline. All the results of the study were also achieved without increases in insulin dose or body weight. A key conclusion of the study was that DIY APS requires learning and involvement from both patients and physicians. The most important conclusion may have been that experience and patience from all parties are needed to become proficient in using the system over time. The limitations of the study include lack of randomized controls, as this was a study done to assess safety. The sample size was also small due to rigorous exclusion criteria as well as lack of reimbursement of CGM devices in the country the study was conducted (Poland). The careful monitoring from highly motivated patients, research team, and support from device company representatives make replication of the study in the real world difficult. Another part of the study that may not be reproducible is the frequency of follow-up and interventions based on the follow-ups [4].

In Lenka Petruzelkova et al. they conducted a randomized trial called Pancreas4ALL in which they studied the safety and viability of the open-source automated insulin delivery via AndroidAPS and compared the effectiveness in three groups: (1) full closed loop (FCL), (2) meal announcement only (MA), and (3) hybrid closed loop with meal bolus (HCL) among adolescents and young adults with type 1 diabetes. There were a total of 16 participants in the study from the age range of 15–20 years old. Other inclusion criteria for the participants were that they had a diagnosis of type 1 diabetes for at least 1 year, they used a CGM and insulin pump for at least 3 months, their HbA1c values were between 6.1% for 43 mmol/mol and 9.7% for 75 mmol/mol, and lastly an agreement to use the automated insulin delivery system continuously throughout the study. Pregnancy and any concurrent medication that affects glucose control were in the exclusion criteria. The participants were from Children Diabetes Center of Motol University Hospital in the Czech Republic. The equipment given to the participants and needed for the study was a Samsung phone with the Pancreas4ALL app, insulin pump DANA RS, and CGM Dexcom G6. The study lasted 10 days—one day of a run-in phase afterward there was a 3-day HCL phase and two 3-day scenarios (MA or FCL) that were randomly assigned. This is the first randomized experiment that assessed the AndroidAPS algorithm, an open-source automated insulin delivery system, in several contexts, including the FCL. Throughout the course of the study, the percentage of time spent in hypoglycemia of less than 54 mg/dL did not exceed 1%. The HCL scenario had a higher percentage that was 1.05%, MA group was 0% and FCL was 0%, with a statistically significant p value = 0.05. The amount of time spent in hypoglycemia between 54 mg/dL and 68.5 mg/dL throughout the course of the day did not change across the three groups (was not statistically significant). All three groups showed good time in range (HCL 82.88% vs. MA 79.85% vs. FCL 81.03%; $p = 0.58$) was demonstrated in all evaluated groups of the Pancreas4ALL system. This is consistent with mean glycemia of 124 mg/dL in the HCL group, 132 mg/dL in the MA group, and 127.3 mg/dL in the FCL group ($p = 0.28$). The participants answered the closed-loop experience questionnaire and in every test context, the participants appreciated the automatic control of their blood glucose; during the FCL, they devoted the least amount of time controlling their diabetes. It's interesting to note that during the HCL scenario, participants exhibited less anxiety about diabetes than they did during the MA and FCL. Additionally, participants reported improvements in the quality of life and diabetes-related symptoms ($p < 0.01$). No difference was seen in TTD (total daily insulin dose) or in the daily carbohydrate intake in all three groups. Throughout this RCT, there were no adverse events. This study showed that the AndroidAPS was able to achieve good glucose management without limiting the amount of carbohydrates consumed, elevating the daily insulin dosage, or spending an inordinate amount of time in hypoglycemia. A few of the study's drawbacks included prolonged hyperglycemia following cannula malfunction, postprandial hyperglycemia in the FCL group when the premeal glucose was less than 72.06 mg/dL or if the participant exercised before a meal, and the fact that the amount of insulin delivered by supermicroboluses is highly dependent on the proper insulin ratio and the insulin sensitivity factor. Some limitations of the study were small sample size and short time period. One of the study's strengths was it was randomized trial design, which included multiple intervention groups, including the full close loop (FCL). Additionally, the research demonstrated the value of performing randomized controlled trials (RCTs) to address potential issues and difficulties that users may run into when utilizing DIY automated insulin delivery systems [5].

Conclusion

The birth and rapid development of DIYAPS is an excellent example of need driving innovation in medical technology. The rapidity of the development has created a lag between regulatory board approval and physician acceptance. The widespread use of DIY technologies within the T1D community, recent FDA approvals of the TidePool application, and various artificial pancreas systems show a promising trend. Continued voluntary sharing of data and creation of new devices will only further enhance these devices that have the potential to improve quality of life and patient safety.

References

1. Kesavadev J, Srinivasan S, Saboo B, Krishna BM, Krishnan G. The do-it-yourself artificial pancreas: a comprehensive review. Diabetes Ther. 2020;11:1217–35.
2. Lewis D. History and perspective on DIY closed looping. J Diabetes Sci Technol. 2019;13(4):790–3.
3. Crabtree TS, McLay A, Wilmot EG. DIY artificial pancreas systems: here to stay? Pract Diabetes. 2019;36(2):63–8.
4. Gawrecki A, Zozulinska-Ziolkiewicz D, Michalak MA, Adamska A, Michalak M, Frackowiak U, Flotynska J, Pietrzak M, Czapla S, Gehr B, Araszkiewicz A. Safety and glycemic outcomes of do-it-yourself AndroidAPS hybrid closed-loop system in adults with type 1 diabetes. PLoS One. 2021;16(4):e0248965. https://doi.org/10.1371/journal.pone.0248965.
5. Petruzelkova L, Neuman V, Plachy L, Kozak M, Obermannova B, Kolouskova S, et al. First use of open-source automated insulin delivery AndroidAPS in full closed-loop scenario: Pancreas4ALL randomized pilot study. Diabetes Technol Ther. 2023;25(5):315–23.

Chapter 9
A Historic FDA Clearance: Open Source Software and the Making of Tidepool Loop

Paige Edmiston

Introduction

On January 24, 2023, the U.S. Food and Drug Administration (FDA) announced the clearance of Tidepool Loop, an automated insulin dosing app. When a medical device is cleared for use, discussions about the new product's significance tend to revolve around how it stacks up, clinically and technologically, to preexisting therapeutic options. Much of the discussion following Tidepool Loop's regulatory clearance has followed a similar blueprint [1, 2]. As important as its novel features may be, however, Tidepool Loop's importance exceeds the app itself. This chapter argues that the technology's larger significance lies in how it was made.[1] Through an anthropological look inside the making of Tidepool Loop—the first fully interoperable, open source diabetes technology to achieve FDA clearance—this chapter offers a primer on what open source means, how it emerged as a solution to key challenges facing software developers, and what it looks like to develop open source software. Finally, drawing on interviews with the developers of Tidepool Loop, this chapter considers pressing challenges facing regulators in the contemporary era of software development and explores the potential role open source could play in the future of medical software.

As a technical approach to software development that unfolds behind-the-scenes, the use of open versus proprietary software development methods is likely to fade undetected into the background of most clinical discussions about diabetes

[1] Tidepool Loop is "fully interoperable" in the sense that it is cleared to work with "third party" (i.e., made by another company) component devices [3, 4].

P. Edmiston (✉)
University of Colorado at Boulder, Boulder, CO, USA
e-mail: paige.edmiston@colorado.edu

S. Fishman (ed.), *Advances in Diabetes Technology*, Contemporary Endocrinology, https://doi.org/10.1007/978-3-031-75352-7_9

technology. But as the stories in this account will suggest, the processes companies use to make software matter, not just at the individual product level but for how medical software operates as a system [5]. Through its very existence as an FDA-cleared alternative to proprietary software, Tidepool Loop proves that developing interoperable, open source software is possible within the health care environment. The larger significance of Tidepool Loop thus lies in the techno-legal reform it signals is possible for computing and regulation in the medical space.

Open Source Software

Open source is a term that is often used and rarely defined. At its simplest, the term "open source" describes software with source code that is made publicly available. Not all source code published publicly on the internet, however, is open source. Though open source projects can vary substantially in purpose, philosophy, governance, and organizational form, they are united by their use of private legal mechanisms to ensure the permissive use of code in the future, thereby enabling a more collaborative "borrow and share" model of software development [6–8]. Methodologically, developing open source software is similar to working with text in Google Docs. Contributors can see the text (or code), suggest edits, and trace what changes were made by whom. They can even copy the text and move it to a different document. But only the people with editing permissions (like the document's owner) can incorporate suggested revisions into the original document (or project, in the case of open source software).[2]

Though open source software development is an outlier in the diabetes device industry, it is the diabetes device industry's closed proprietary approach that is the outlier in the wider world of contemporary software development. Open source software can be created through bottom-up, user-led community projects. But it is not exclusive to grassroots projects. It is also used, developed, and organized by some of the world's largest technology companies, including Google, Amazon, and Microsoft. As one Tidepool developer explained to me, "In the last decade, open source has changed from being something that's more niche to just almost the way that software is written now."[3]

Open source is perhaps best understood in relation to its opposite. Contrary to popular assumptions, proprietary and open source software are not divided by commercial-noncommercial, professional-volunteer, or regulated-unregulated lines. The key difference is techno-legal. Where open source licenses invert the

[2] I thank Christopher Snider for this insight.

[3] Open source software development is also distinct from the concept of interoperability—though, as this chapter will explore, the historical impetus for open source was, in part, the problem of interoperability. To be clear, open source software development is not the only solution to the problem of interoperability, and proprietary software can be made to be interoperable. Nor is interoperability the only reason an organization might choose to use open source methods.

traditional function of copyrights—with the copyright holders exercising their exclusive rights not to restrict code but, rather, to liberate it—proprietary software is developed under licensing agreements that restrict the distribution, use, and modification of source code. The distinction is also rooted in different cultural ideas about economic value. Where proprietary approaches believe the value of code to lie in its secrecy, open software advocates believe making source code freely available leads to higher quality software overall [7].

Within the diabetes technology literature, discussion of open source has largely focused on the experiences of people in the do-it-yourself (DIY) diabetes community who have used open source code to build their own remote monitoring software and insulin dosing apps at home. In this literature, DIY and open source are often used interchangeably, likely because, until recently, the highest profile open source diabetes software required users to build their own systems. However, as open source systems have emerged that do not require users to build the systems themselves, the conflation of these terms has led to confusion.

Take, for instance, the results of the CREATE (Community Derived Automated Insulin Delivery) trial published in the *New England Journal of Medicine*, which evaluated the effectiveness of an automated insulin delivery (AID) system developed through an open source community project [9]. Reflecting upon reactions to the trial, Dana Lewis, one of the study's co-authors and a well-known DIY advocate, observed in a blog post how the popular conflation of DIY and open source led to misunderstandings. "One area that I've noticed is frequently misunderstood is how 'open source' and 'DIY' are different…You can DIY with open source. But open source and DIY are not the same thing" [10]. Though the technology investigated in this trial was open source and had for many years been available for people to build themselves, the devices and software used in the study were not DIY. Participants were provided a pre-built device, meaning they did not have to follow instructions or use code to build their own systems [10]. This study was designed to evaluate the safety and efficacy of an app and algorithm developed through an open source project community, not (in this case) to study DIY practices specifically.[4] As open source diabetes technologies emerge that have achieved FDA clearance and do not require users to build the devices themselves, it is worth asking: When analytically cleaved from DIY, does a company's choice to employ open

[4] By insisting on the distinction between open source and DIY, I do not mean to distance open source diabetes technology from the DIY community, nor to discount the critical role DIY users have played in many of today's open source projects (including Tidepool Loop). Instead, I mean to point out that the relationship between open source and DIY in diabetes technology is historically contingent, not inherent. It is also not to say DIY projects lack governance (as discussed later in this chapter) or evidence. Numerous observational studies have examined the clinical effectiveness and quality of life of people who build their own systems, including cross-disciplinary research by an EU-funded research consortium called the OPEN Project [11–17]. The 2023 ADA Standards of Care also provided guidance to clinicians on the use of DIY systems.

source or proprietary software development practice matter to clinicians and patients?[5]

Using Tidepool Loop as a case study, this chapter considers whether and how the conditions and practices shaping the development of software matter to clinicians and patients. Tidepool Loop is an open source—but not DIY—mobile app. The app will be available for download from the App Store like any other iOS app.[6] Drawing on original interviews with 17 people involved in the making of Tidepool Loop and an analysis of publicly available documents and media,[7] this account historicizes the making of Tidepool Loop, situating its production in the broader cultural phenomenon of open source. It also offers an anthropological window into the benefits, challenges, practicalities, and possibilities of open source from the perspective of the people behind the first FDA-cleared, open source, and fully interoperable diabetes technology.

What follows is the story of how Tidepool Loop came to be.

The Problem with Proprietary Software

Since the earliest days of computers, computer scientists have dreamed of The Computer—a universal machine capable of performing any calculation using any data. But, as anthropologist Christopher Kelty puts it, "we do not live in the world of The Computer—we live in a world of *computers*" ([21], p. 121). Anyone who has wished to use an app made only for a different operating system—or spent precious time scrolling through an unorganized dump of scanned documents from another health system's electronic health record—has encountered the problem of multiple computers. In theory, the solution is simple. Systems can be designed so that information can move freely between various devices. But in practice, this technological ideal—the free and seamless exchange of data across computers—has long existed in tension with an economic and legal intellectual property system that encourages secrecy and jealous ownership ([21], p. 144). When developers fail to collaborate—through sharing code and agreeing to standards—users can find

[5] To date, social scientific research on open source diabetes technologies has also tended to focus on its DIY applications. Focusing on the practices and politics of DIY, social scientists have argued that these patient-led technological interventions represent a potential realignment of the traditional dynamics of power and expertise in doctor–patient and manufacturer–user relationships [18, 19]. By situating Tidepool Loop in a larger cultural and professional history of software development, this chapter considers how foregrounding open source practices might shed light on how two "competing regimes of expertise"—information technology and medicine—negotiate their cultural differences amidst the digital transformation of health care, as software increasingly becomes the medium through which health care happens ([20], p. 645).

[6] Tidepool Loop is an iOS app. The company plans to release an Android version in the future. See "Things you should know": https://www.tidepool.org/tidepool-loop

[7] Following anthropological conventions, my research participants are not identified by name, except in the case of well-known figures in the diabetes community whose names have been used with their permission. The research for this chapter was conducted with approval from the University of Colorado Boulder IRB and supported by a National Science Foundation Graduate Research Fellowship.

themselves "trapped" in proprietary systems, stripped of choice and unable to move (their data) between systems and devices.

The problem of multiple computers was top of mind for a group of software developers and entrepreneurs gathered in a small Stanford University conference room in the fall of 2013. At this first D-Data Exchange, a now annual event that convenes patients, entrepreneurs, regulators, and industry leaders to discuss the development of data-driven technologies for diabetes, participants included future leaders of well-known open source projects, like the Nightscout Foundation, OpenAPS, and Tidepool, and companies like Dexcom, Glooko, Beta Bionics, and Bigfoot Biomedical [22]. This, however, was still 2013. Some of these organizations were in their infancy; others yet to be formed. Yet to the people gathered in the room that day, one thing was clear: the state of diabetes technology was unacceptable. Summarizing this sentiment, Lane Desborough, a "geek dad" of a child with diabetes (who went on to play a key role in the Nightscout Foundation, among other projects) threw out a theme. With little sense of what this slogan would one day become, Howard Look, founder and CEO of the (then) newly formed Tidepool, jotted Desborough's phrase—"we are not waiting"—on the white board, later tweeting it from the Tidepool account. This tweet is believed to be the first use of the #wearenotwaiting hashtag, a slogan that was widely taken up by DIY diabetes projects around the world in the years that followed. One month after the D-Data Exchange, Tidepool published a guest post titled "We Are Not Waiting," in which Desborough summarized the session's takeaways:

> Companies that make physical components of (the diabetes) ecosystem...will continue to survive and thrive because these elements are necessary... What will change is how—and how fast—these systems will be developed. Closed, proprietary systems will die. Open, standards-based, interoperable devices will thrive...We are not waiting [22].

From today's vantage point, where multiple commercial (and at least partially interoperable) automated insulin dosing (AID) systems are now commercially available, this statement may appear unexceptional. But a decade ago, when this post was published, the diabetes technology market was dominated by one giant corporation. Because hardware and software were bundled, people with diabetes wearing pumps had to wait until they were eligible to get a new physical device (typically 4 or 5 years) to access any software updates.[8] Continuous glucose monitors were still 3 years away from being cleared by the FDA to make diabetes treatment decisions [24]. No open source AID systems were yet in development. Commercial systems were even further away. Not everyone thought this—the use of proprietary software and its relationship to the state of diabetes technology—was a problem. For many, it was normalized. This was simply how diabetes technology worked. But for a group of people gathered in Stanford conference room on a fall day in 2013, the problem of closed, proprietary software appeared self-evident.

We might attribute the obviousness of the problem to the personal, first-hand experiences with type 1 diabetes that united many of the people in the room that day.

[8] In 2017, Tandem Diabetes Care became the first company to enable software updates for insulin pumps using a personal computer [23].

When asked to explain their involvement with #wearenotwaiting, community members often point to their personal stories with diabetes. Take, for example, the story Howard Look tells about the inspiration for Tidepool in a public interview with diabetes blogger Kerri Sparling [25]. When his elementary-age daughter was diagnosed with type 1 diabetes, tracking glucose and insulin data became a routine part of his family's life. Yet despite this directive to care for numbers, the devices and software available at the time did not allow people to simultaneously view data from the various devices they relied upon, even at the doctor's office. When we spoke, Look recalled an example. "I literally once saw an endocrinologist hold the printouts [of various data reports] up to the light and try to lay them on top of each other to see if we could line data up that way, which of course didn't work. That was the beginning of my personal frustration. Why is it so hard to see the data from my daughter's devices and get her the best possible care?"

As a long-time professional in the software industry (including leadership roles at Amazon, TiVo, and Pixar), Look was well acquainted with what modern software could do. In comparison, he likened his attempts to access his daughter's device data to "crawling through glass" [26]. In the interview with Sparling [25], Look described his early efforts to access his daughter's data:

> I won't call it hacking. Compared to what other people in the DIY community did, what I did was slightly technical nudging. I made it so we could see [my daughter's CGM and pump data] in one place. I was like, why isn't anyone doing anything about this? As a geek dad, I tried to find other people who were thinking like I was and, to make a long story short, I ended up founding Tidepool because of that.

As the parent of a daughter with diabetes, Look was intimately familiar with and motivated to address the frustrations diabetes posed in everyday life. But this fact, on its own, cannot explain why he arrived at the dominance of closed, proprietary companies within the diabetes technology space—and their restrictive approach to data access—as the problem in need of solving. Lots of people, after all, have diabetes (or children with diabetes) and many have found themselves frustrated with their devices or data. But in 2013, few found the state of diabetes technology as peculiar—and as obviously solvable—as did the group of people gathered for the first D-Data Exchange. As Look explained to Sparling, he was a "geek dad." His expectations for software reflected his social location as a professional working in the technology space, as well as the burgeoning movement for "data liberation" unfolding in health technology circles at the time.[9] For geeks working in Silicon

---

[9] As this example illustrates, foregrounding patient identities or professional expertise shifts the narrative of #wearenotwaiting, leading to distinct (though not incompatible) interpretations of the movement's significance. By highlighting the personal diabetes stories and DIY practices of those involved, #wearenotwaiting becomes a powerful story of patient activism and bottom-up innovation that challenges traditional categories and hierarchies of expertise. At the same time, by foregrounding its early members' "geek" identities, #wearenotwaiting fits into the larger story of health care's digital transformation, providing a glimpse into how software professionals interpreted the problems facing medical technology. This period also coincides with the first Health Datapalooza and the entry of the "data liberation" movement into health care and technology circles [27].

Valley in the 2010s, the state of diabetes technology was bewildering precisely because the problem it faced, in their estimation, had already been solved by modern software development techniques and processes.

The computing industry's first large-scale attempt to solve the problem of interoperability came in the 1980s when software was, for the first time, de-bundled from hardware [6, 21]. The "open systems" approach aimed to create "seamless integration" for users. If all participants were to adopt the same design of systems, the thinking went, it would "lead to widely interoperable, integrated machines that could send, store, process, and receive the user's information" ([21], p. 147). Its success required the standardization of computing infrastructure which, in turn, hinged on building a consensus among stakeholders—an attempt that ultimately proved fruitless. By the end of the decade, proprietary computing had reasserted its dominance in the form of Microsoft Windows ([21], p. 164). With no clear financial incentives, the open systems experiment failed to get investors and corporations to collaborate, each vying with the other to set and control the standards. The necessary economic model did not exist—at least, not yet.[10]

Then, in the 1990s, a counterintuitive solution to the tension between intellectual property and interoperability emerged. Originating in academic computer science departments, the free software movement tackled the problem of collaboration by "hacking" copyright law. Taking advantage of the strong intellectual property rights granted by federal law, this hack used property rights to "actually loosen the restrictions normally associated with ownership" ([21], p. 182). Unlike the public domain, where material (like code) is made freely usable without restriction, free software licenses used the restrictions granted to the rights holder to "free" their code from restrictions [8]. Under free software licenses, code is permitted for use by anybody for any purpose *so long as they in turn attach the same restriction*, thereby protecting all future uses of the code from restriction. As free software advocates quip, free software is free like speech, not beer [34]. Free, in other words, is not about cost but refers instead to a particular conception of liberty where code is understood, like speech, to be subject to certain freedoms.

By the end of the decade, there emerged an ideological fork in the free software world between free software and open source. Though free software and open source practices, licenses, and organizational forms were (at the time) essentially identical, their respective advocates argued fiercely over the purpose of "freeing" software. Where free software advocates were explicitly political, positioning free

[10] This story may sound familiar to clinicians working in the twenty-first century. Electronic health record companies like Cerner and Epic have similarly attempted to create "openness" by imposing their own "interoperability networks," an experiment that has resulted in a patchwork system rather than the seamless exchange of medical records envisioned by the HITECH Act [28]. Notably, SMART by FHIR, an open source, standards-based API for EHRs, has been adopted in recent years by some of the largest EHR vendors; its use is required by health information technologies certified by the Office of the National Coordinator for Health Information Technology (ONC) [29, 30]. Similar efforts to establish open standards are ongoing among diabetes software developers [31]. Open source and open standards are distinct but related approaches to tackling the issue of interoperability [32, 33].

software as an issue of freedom of expression and self-determination, open source advocates were zealously pragmatic. Downplaying the free software movement's philosophical and political claims, open source advocates emphasized the practical superiority of open source over proprietary approaches to software development, promising business leaders "better quality, higher reliability, more flexibility, lower cost, and an end to predatory vendor lock-in" ([8], p. 30). Contrary to Microsoft's early 2000s accusations of "communism," neither free software nor open source advocates were anti-commercial [35]. Both groups understood themselves as reformists, aiming to "save capitalism from the capitalists"—like Microsoft—who they believed were stifling innovation and constricting consumer choice ([21], p. 71). But where free software advocates foregrounded free software as a "social movement," concerned first and foremost with the preservation of "freedom," open source advocates highlighted its pragmatism as a software development methodology, seeking to make open source more attractive to business [8, 36].

By the first decade of the twenty-first century, open source advocates had succeeded. Open source projects became the foundation of "the cloud" [37]. Microsoft—the corporation most famously opposed to open source —came to embrace it, even buying GitHub (a major hub for the open source community) in 2018 [38, 39]. Like Amazon and Google, Microsoft's contributions to and investment in open source projects have only continued to grow. To be clear, open source did not bring about the world of The Computer. Our world today is a world of "platforms." Android apps, for example, do not work on Apple phones. Nor do issues of data access, interoperability, and open source perfectly map onto one another. As Look explained, "You could have a liberal view of data access and still be closed, proprietary, and you could be open source and still not have a right to access data view." But open source, as a techno-legal model of software development, did change how people expect to interact with data, devices, and software. And perhaps most importantly, it changed how software developers expected to be able to work. Open source not only created the conditions for interoperability, it also saved developers from "having to rebuild the same damn thing over and over again" [37]. For companies and other software projects, this meant more time to focus on the problem at hand rather than having to solve problems that had already been solved. As one software developer at Tidepool explained to me:

> By using open source we can benefit from literally hundreds of years of work that others have done. Our mission is to spend our time building software that helps with diabetes, so we should not go and build the next service deployment tool or a compiler or a fancy way of rendering some user interface on a web form or something like that. We would much rather leverage existing solutions for that as opposed to building, spending our precious resources building those things because someone has already built them...We are standing on the shoulders of giants and combined we can become a lot taller all together.

Open source saved companies (and developers) from having to continuously reinvent the wheel, from having to build (or buy) their own service deployment tools and compilers, creating shorter, less expensive production cycles, and avoiding duplicated efforts. Through open source projects, large corporations have not only collaborated with startups, universities, and government organizations, but they have also found ways to work with their competitors in the marketplace ([6], p. 40). By creating the conditions for collaboration, open source freed consumers from becoming trapped in closed, proprietary systems (albeit not to the extent that free software advocates had hoped).

By the time "geeks" like Look encountered diabetes devices in early 2010s, open source had already gone mainstream. It was not just an economic model or development method. It had become a cultural ideal, widely understood among a generation of software developers as the "obvious" way to build software. In their professional milieu, it was simply the way "good" software was made.[11] The state of diabetes technology, in contrast, was experienced as a kind of temporal "culture shock"—a jarring return (to borrow one interview subject's description of the diabetes device industry at the time) to the "dark ages" of computing when corporate "overlords" locked people and their data into substandard systems. While it was perplexing, if not shocking, that such a problem existed at all, for geeks working in information technology in the mid-2010s, the path to modernization would have been clear. It was, after all, a familiar problem with an existing solution. Desborough's forecast—that closed, proprietary system would "die" while open, interoperable devices would "thrive"—was as much a geek's reading of the past as it was a diabetes parent's prediction for the future. "We are not waiting" was a call to bring an outdated diabetes device industry into the software of the present—not just in product but in practice.

Open Source Branches

Though early members of the #wearenotwaiting community agreed that closed, proprietary systems were the problem and open, interoperable systems were the solution, how precisely to go about developing open systems remained a question mark. Contrary to popular narrations of open source as almost magically self-organizing, open source projects require organizational structure. And like most collaborative endeavors, starting, leading, growing, and maintaining a successful open source project requires labor, as well good governance and diplomacy [34]. To shed light on how open source works in practice, I trace two branches of the #wearenotwaiting trunk, Tidepool and DIY Loop, and how the crossing of their respective paths made possible the first-ever clearance of an open source diabetes device.[12] Together, these two branches provide a glimpse into the everyday work and organizational heterogeneity of open source software development.

[11] Look cites Mozilla, Android, Second Life (by Linden Lab), and Linux as sources of inspiration for adopting an open source approach.

[12] In software development, a "branch" refers to an "independent line of development" [40]. Unlike a "fork" (a discrete copy of a project), the code developed in a branch can be merged back into the main project or "trunk."

Branch-Tidepool

In 2011, Brandon Arbiter was living in New York City, leading business intelligence and data management for an online grocery company. To help the company make "data-driven decisions" about, for example, late delivery issues, Arbiter built systems to integrate different data sources. "You've got a stream of data from this system, and a stream of data from that system…You need to put those together to see how late deliveries are happening."

That same year, he found out he had type 1 diabetes.

"I got an insulin pump put on me. I got a glucose monitor put on me," Arbiter recalled during our video call, rolling up his t-shirt sleeves to show me his devices, one attached to each arm. In the days following his diagnosis, Arbiter scoured the internet in search of software that could integrate the data from his pump and monitor. "There was no software on the planet where you could take the data from these devices and look at them together. This was the same exact problem that I solved every day at work…It was unbelievable [that the software didn't already exist]. And so, I did it myself." Though he did not yet know it, Arbiter was not alone in his disbelief over the state of diabetes technology.

After sharing his initial work online, Arbiter was introduced to Howard Look by a mutual connection. United by their frustration over the "sorry state of diabetes technology," Arbiter and Look hit it off, though each had a different idea for how to proceed. Where Arbiter envisioned a specific software application that would combine and use glucose, insulin, and meal information to create personalized recommendations, Look wanted to tackle the problem of data access directly. Arbiter had arrived at a fork in the road: pursue his idea or join Look's nascent organization. "Ultimately, I thought, if we build an open data platform that actually solves the problem that is preventing me from doing what I want to do—there are probably a lot of other people trying to innovate that have the same problem. So, I dropped what I wanted to do, left my job in New York, and moved out to join Howard."

In September 2013, a few months before the first D-Data Exchange, Arbiter arrived in California, ready to begin work on Tidepool. The founding team wanted Tidepool to be everything the diabetes device industry was not. Where diabetes technology was built by "stodgy old-school companies," they would be a tech-forward nonprofit [41]. Instead of "closed, proprietary systems…[that] hoard the data generated by their device," Tidepool would be open source and open data [41]. They wanted to create a space where researchers and entrepreneurs could innovate and collaborate, and where people with diabetes could upload, view, and interact with their data regardless of the device that generated it. But figuring out what it meant to be "open" was itself an experiment. "We said we were open source. We said we were open data," Arbiter recalled. "But we didn't truly understand what all that meant at the beginning."

In the beginning, Look and Arbiter envisioned Tidepool as an open source project community where people would not just download code but contribute it as well, drawing on one of the most tantalizing and romanticized potential outcomes of open source—that is, coordinating a far-flung community of individual contributors around a shared goal. In practice, accepting external contributions proved too expensive. "It would be like three weeks of work on our part to get one day of work out of some third-party individual," Arbiter told me. This realization became a "forcing function" for Tidepool. In user experience design, a forcing function is an element of design that compels the user to consciously (rather than passively) consider the choice before them. These unanticipated costs forced early Tidepool team members to thoughtfully revisit why they were open source, if not to attract external contributions. "There were still plenty of reasons…That would have been awesome [to accept outside contributions] but that was the least important reason among them," Arbiter reflected.

When I asked other Tidepool team members to explain the value of open source, several offered a similar example. As one developer exclaimed, "I've seen screenshots of the Tidepool Uploader in German. I'm like, wow, this is so cool!" Not just in Germany, but developers in Denmark, France, Colombia, and elsewhere had copied and modified Tidepool's data platform to create similar products localized to their respective national and language markets [42, 43]. As a small nonprofit with limited resources, open source licenses enabled Tidepool's technology to potentially reach users, like those in other countries, they would not be able to reach on their own. In an industry built on proprietary models where value lies in secrecy, this celebration of seeing one's intellectual property used freely by others can seem counterintuitive. Yet this inversion—where seeing one's code copied and modified is transformed from a property violation to a sign of success—is part of the cleverness of open source as a legal hack [34]. Free and open source licenses enabled a new economic model that—unlike proprietary software which incentivizes isolated development to preserve secrecy—encouraged developers to "borrow and share" [6].

Not all open source users will become contributors but the nature of software incentivizes contributions back to the project. Unlike hardware, which is more stable in form, software is in a perpetual state of change. Sharing new features or bug fixes back to "the community or project that created the original software borrowed ensures easier engineering access to the new and fixed functionality on a go-forward basis" ([6], p. 38). Companies that use open source software without contributing may find the software they incorporated into their project proceeded in directions incompatible with their own. There is, as one developer explained to me, a collective benefit to teams that choose to collaborate:

> We've made [the source code] available for others and in turn those people and teams have contributed their localized versions back to us. We're sort of in this iterative improvement. We provide something of value to them, they provide that to us, and we roll it forward, pay it forward. Alone it would take us years to get there, but with these other folks out there doing some of that work, the overall lift becomes lighter.

This production model differs substantially from the traditional approach to device development employed by the medical technology industry. Usually when a device company wants to launch a new product, they analyze the existing marketplace and aim to launch something entirely different from what already exists.

"We're like no, no, no—start with what we've done and then just make it better. Focus on taking things to the next level," Arbiter told me. "We're trying to create a space where other people don't have to worry about stepping on our toes…which is a different mindset." The goal was not just to reach users in other markets. It was also to change the device landscape in which Tidepool operated.

There was one just one problem. To show the big companies that developing an open, interoperable diabetes, data platform was possible, they first had to convince those very same companies—companies rooted in a very different techno-legal and economic model—to share data with Tidepool. "People thought it was crazy that we were going to go negotiate all these device deals," Arbiter recalled. At the time, many device manufacturers had "fantasies about data as the new oil" ([44], p. 41). From the manufacturers' perspective, device data was "their" data. It did not belong to the people whose bodies generated it. Within several years, however, Tidepool had established contracts with nearly all the major diabetes device manufacturers. Not every company came to the table, but many did. At the time of writing, Tidepool's data platform supports dozens of devices, including glucose monitors, meters, pumps, and pens.

One developer attributed Tidepool's negotiating success to the organization's nonprofit structure. "When Howard created the company, he made it very wisely as a nonprofit. I think that's allowed us to create connections and relationships with other for-profit companies…If we were for-profit, we might be competitors, but because we are nonprofit, I think it's easier to see us collaborators," he said. In an industry of competitors, Tidepool's nonprofit status signaled their neutrality. By shifting liability from an individual to a legally recognizable entity, their legal structure also made their work legible to institutions like the FDA in a way that unincorporated open source project communities—composed of individuals—were not.

Branch-DIY-Loop

While Tidepool was getting off the ground, Pete Schwamb was learning firsthand about diabetes. In 2013, Schwamb's 6-year-old daughter, Riley, was diagnosed with type 1 diabetes. When Riley first started wearing a CGM and insulin pump, Schwamb—a software engineer by trade—began investigating what he could do with her data to help improve her glucose levels and make this new part of their family, diabetes, easier to manage for everyone. "It was pretty much all-consuming," he recalled during our interview. "You're up all the time. You're always checking the numbers. And it was a real pain having to ask Riley for her numbers. She was six years old and running around. Every time I asked, she was completely annoyed." Like Look, Schwamb found the process of accessing Riley's data from her devices unnecessarily difficult. "I was a software engineer and—I could barely do it," he told me, still incredulous 8 years later. "I was like, nobody else is going to be able to do this, so no one is really looking at their data. No one [truly] has access to their data. That was probably when I first [realized] there might be other people interested in this kind of thing."

From Twitter, Schwamb learned about a group on Gitter, a chat platform for software developers where other people with personal connections to diabetes were venting about similar frustrations and sharing hacks. Through this group, Schwamb met some of the early developers involved with Nightscout, an open source, DIY project developing software to remotely monitor glucose levels. This technology was developed by and for parents, like Schwamb, who wanted to keep track of their child's glucose without having to look directly at the device attached to their child's body [45, 46].[13] Schwamb jumped into the conversation to share what he had been working on: a little device that would allow a person's phone and insulin pump, which "speak" different languages, to "talk" to one another. He called the device the "RileyLink."

The RileyLink was a personal hack—a workaround—that allowed Schwamb, who wanted to see the patterns in his daughter's glucose numbers, to access the data on his daughter's device. Nate Racklyeft, another person in the chat room, had a different idea about how the RileyLink could be used. Racklyeft had been working on an algorithm to control his own insulin delivery, and the RileyLink promised to provide the missing link, allowing Racklyeft's mobile app to communicate with and command his insulin pump [48]. Schwamb was not so sure:

> I was actually not that interested in the automation part. I was interested in getting the data. I don't think I realized the impact that automation can have—and it was also kind of scary. All this stuff has bugs. I know that my software has bugs. I know that everybody's software has bugs. The idea of making a piece of software that was controlling insulin delivery was pretty freaky at that time. It's crazy how we talk about it now…But back then, it was even more…Just talking about it seemed some kind of crazy, right?

Around this time, another member of the chat room had started assembling RileyLinks using Schwamb's designs and shipping them to those in the community who wanted to use them. Each board could take hours to make. Racklyeft received one of the boards from the first shipment of RileyLinks, which he used to start making what would eventually become DIY Loop. He had DIY Loop up and running (on himself) by early 2016. By this point, Schwamb had started to see the automation of insulin delivery as a "potentially really powerful thing." But still, he was hesitant to have Riley use it. "When Nate said he had it running, I didn't start it right then. I actually waited a bit." Eventually, Pete and his wife decided to try it. "We had to run it while watching it every minute basically to see what it was doing. But it was really quick after seeing it work and seeing it adjust things to [realize]—oh my gosh, we could actually be sleeping and it's just doing its thing."

I clarified. "That was running with…Riley was using it?"

---

[13] Dana Lewis, Scott Leibrand, and Ben West's respective work on OpenAPS, the first open source and DIY "artificial pancreas" project, also played a critical role in laying the groundwork for DIY Loop [47]. Illustrating the interconnectedness of these various projects, the pump that West first reverse engineered was Arbiter's pump. Arbiter and West were roommates when Arbiter first moved to California.

"Yeah, right. My daughter Riley was using it. So, you know, I was staying up and watching it as she slept making sure it was doing what we expected it to do."

The system worked beautifully, reading Riley's glucose levels and adjusting how and when her pump delivered insulin accordingly.

Later that same year, Racklyeft had to step away from his work on DIY Loop. He asked Schwamb to take over as the project lead. I asked Schwamb if taking on the role was a hard decision. It was, after all, a lot of time and responsibility. In just a few years, thousands of people would rely on the DIY Loop code to build their own automated insulin dosing systems. It wasn't a hard decision, he told me. In fact, Schwamb explained, it didn't feel like a decision at all. "[DIY Loop] is transformative in terms of quality of life—being able to sleep through the night and all that.... I still had a full-time job and was busy...but this was obviously something that was really important, so I never really questioned whether or not it was an option to not do so."

Schwamb was not the only parent to find DIY Loop transformative. Like many "Loopers" (people using DIY Loop), Katie DiSimone—whose daughter also lives with type 1—first learned about DIY Loop on the internet, where she stumbled upon an Instagram post depicting a child holding an iPhone with the caption: "First day back at school. Using Loop to control type 1. This is amazing. Thanks!" Writing in 2023, the idea of using a phone to automate insulin delivery no longer seems outlandish, but in 2016 it was, in DiSimone's words, "shocking." Through the post, she found the Gitter chat group where people (like Schwamb) were discussing DIY Loop. Members of the chat directed her to the project's public website where there were instructions, written by the project's developers, for how to build DIY Loop.

A civil engineer by trade, DiSimone was skilled in working through problems methodically. Having previously built a mobile app from a template before, she also had cursory knowledge of what the process entailed. Curious and hopeful, DiSimone decided to try building DIY Loop, following the instructions in the public Google Doc. The first step went smoothly. Then, DiSimone hit a roadblock. "When you looked at the 'build the app' instructions, it had a line I will never forget. It said, 'insert meat and potatoes here'." The "meat and potatoes" were the key instructions, and they were missing. She spent a full week experimenting with different permutations. "I just struggled through and didn't give up...Then suddenly one day it was built! It was there on the phone," DiSimone recalled. Her initial excitement was tempered by the realization she had not documented the steps. So, she deleted the app and built it all over again, carefully recording each step.

In the fall of that same year, Nightscout, another open source diabetes project, announced a hackathon in San Francisco where developers from various projects, including DIY Loop, planned to meet. "I was dead set on being there, so I could give them a hug in person and say thank you," DiSimone said. She vividly remembers meeting Schwamb. "I asked him: 'what can I do? You've changed my life! What can I do to repay you?' I remember he looked at me and [said], 'I don't know. You'll find something. You'll find your way [to contribute]." DiSimone spent the rest of the day contemplating how she could give back the project which had already, in the few short months since she built it, transformed her family's life. Eventually, it came to her. She would write out the "meat and potatoes." "I told Pete—I figured it out! I am going to write up the directions [for DIY Loop]. I'm just warning you: you're going to need more RileyLinks. Because when we get done...You don't know how many soccer moms like me are out there, waiting for this. And when they see it's real? It felt like the moment in *Jaws*. 'You're gonna need a bigger boat!'"

Unlike Tidepool, which is structured as a nonprofit and employs developers to create its open source software, DIY Loop's volunteer contributors were not connected through any formal legal structure. However, the absence of legal structure does not mean DIY Loop lacked governance. DIY Loop operates under what open source advocates call a "benevolent dictator model" ([6, 49], p. 54). In this model of open source governance, the "benevolent dictator," or project lead, has the final say over what contributions are merged into the project's software. In DIY's Loop's case, Schwamb is the project lead (having inherited the role from Racklyeft). Though "dictator" implies absolute authority, project leads are accountable to their community. Because open source licenses allow anyone to fork (copy the code and create a competing project), to maintain and grow their project, project leads have to be skilled in diplomacy and responsive to their community members.[14]

To be successful, an open source community project needs to have contributors—that is, community members who build features or fix bugs, among other tasks. A contribution is submitted as a "pull request" which is then reviewed by the project lead to determine whether the pull request will be merged into the project. But people do not have to be software developers to become contributors to open source projects. Contributions can also involve writing documentation or supporting new users who were, in the case of DIY Loop, the people building their own apps at home. In the early days of DIY Loop, contributors and users were largely the same people. DiSimone's prediction, however, proved true. Once the documentation and support was in place, DIY Loop took off.[15] As the DIY Loop community grew, not all users became contributors, though there remained a "pay it forward" ethic. "It is not that people are in or out. It is a huge continuum of involvement with different levels of contribution," Schwamb told me. A large group of people contributed occasionally, offering assistance and mentorship to newer users, for example. It was a much smaller group of core contributors who developed the code and documentation.[16]

As DIY Loop grew in popularity, so too did Schwamb's concerns about liability. One of the challenges of leading unincorporated open source project communities is that, as the project grows, so too does the responsibility placed on the project maintainers ([6], p. 65). The nature of DIY Loop—as a medical device delivering a high-stakes medication—compounded this concern. From the perspective of the

[14] FreeAPS, for example, was a fork of DIY Loop.

[15] Researchers estimate that, as of 2020, thousands of people had built their own DIY Loop [13].

[16] The DIY Loop community lost one of its most dedicated contributors and leaders when Katie DiSimone passed away from glioblastoma in 2023 [50]. The outpouring of support and gratitude from the Looper community throughout DiSimone's cancer journey and following her passing testify to the difference she made in the lives of thousands of people with diabetes and their families.

DIY diabetes community, building one's own medical device was a form of self-experimentation, not commercial activity, excluding it from regulatory purview. As the project leads of OpenAPS, the first open source automated insulin dosing (AID) system, explained on their website, "individuals who build an OpenAPS are essentially doing an (n = 1) experiment, which they have a right to do to/by themselves. That is not a regulated activity by the FDA" [51]. On the DIY Loop website, users encountered a similar disclaimer stating the project's lack of regulatory approval and absolving the project's developers of any responsibility [52].

Nevertheless, the ambiguity of the situation bothered Schwamb. "I had conversations with [people from the FDA] that were sometimes scary because, you know, they obviously believe Loop falls into the category of a regulated device," Schwamb told me. "They wanted a responsible party for this, somebody that's going to stand up and be behind it [if something goes wrong] ...They said they were exercising discretion about it. And so, it was always kind of iffy. I always felt iffy." In the wake of these conversations, Schwamb started pondering how he might transform Loop into a regulated product. Seemingly out of the blue, he received a message from Look.

Tidepool Loop

In April 2018, two of the major diabetes grantmaking foundations hosted a working session to "explore the technical, regulatory and liability landscape for compatible and interoperable Automated Insulin Dosing systems" [53]. Brandon Arbiter, Tidepool's Vice President of Business Development and Strategic Partnerships, set the scene for me: "Howard and I are sitting in the audience, and we can see that the [foundations] are all about interoperability. The CEO of JDRF—at the time, the chief mission officer—was [personally] using DIY Loop...The FDA was talking about interoperability too." During the workshop, an FDA official gave an intriguing presentation, laying out how, theoretically, three device components that did not yet exist—an alternate controller enabled (ACE) pump, an integrated continuous glucose monitor (iCGM), and an interoperable automated glycemic controller (iAGC)—could each be made by different manufacturers and independently reviewed by the FDA. Once cleared, these three components could be used together to create an AID system, distributing responsibility across the different manufacturers according to clearly defined roles. In this theoretical model, consumers would be able to "mix and match" components, picking their preferred pump, monitor, and controller, to create the AID system best suited to their individualized diabetes [54]. In 2018, this pathway was entirely theoretical—no medical device had yet pursued regulatory clearance for an interoperable closed loop system— but it was a pathway nonetheless.[17] Look leaned over to Arbiter while the official talked: "I think we can commercialize Loop."[18]

---

[17] The first hybrid closed-loop system, Medtronic's 670G, was approved under a different regulatory pathway.

[18] This is a recollection from the author's interview with Brandon Arbiter.

In the following weeks, Schwamb received a message. “Let’s talk,” Look wrote to Schwamb. “I’ve got a crazy idea.” Though Schwamb did not know Look personally, he agreed to take the call. While Schwamb and DiSimone had been busy working on DIY Loop, Tidepool had been steadily “freeing” data from commercial diabetes products so that people with diabetes could view and analyze the data from all their devices in one place. Where freeing data using the DIY approach involved reverse engineering—deconstructing how the devices worked (often for purposes other than those intended by the manufacturers)—Tidepool had taken a different approach to interoperability: negotiating contracts and sharing data protocols with the device companies. Collectively, these two branches of #wearenotwaiting had created the technical, relational, and legal components needed to take an open source, AID system through the FDA’s proposed process. DiSimone remembered first hearing about the potential Tidepool-DIY Loop collaboration: “You just get those chills over your body when you know something fits. And that was how it was when I heard Tidepool and Loop might work together. It’s like—wait a second, that would be amazing! It’s a nonprofit, it’s all type-1-centric, these people have skin in the game.”

In October 2018, Tidepool announced their intentions to take Loop through the FDA process, and Schwamb and DiSimone joined the organization as employees. Over the next few years, they developed the technical, legal, and organizational infrastructure and clinical evidence necessary to prove to the FDA that this open source mobile app could be safely and effectively used with component devices to dose insulin—no DIY required. In January 2023, 2 years following their initial 510(k) submission and five years following the announcement of the project, the FDA announced the clearance of Tidepool Loop, the first fully interoperable insulin dosing mobile app, for marketing. By this time, Tidepool Loop was not the first AID system to reach the market. Tandem Control-IQ achieved clearance in 2019 and Omnipod 5 did so in 2022. But it was the first automated glycemic controller cleared to work with any combination of component devices. In so doing, Tidepool Loop materialized the broader “mix and match” vision outlined by the FDA’s regulatory pathway for interoperable AID systems, making it easier (as a “predicate device”) for future developers to also clear products capable of interacting with devices made by other developers.

Open Source for Public Health

“One thing I do think that is kind of a misconception is that the openness and the FDA regulatory side of things are incompatible. In fact, I don’t think that’s at all true,” one Tidepool developer observed to me, during our video call. This developer’s reflection refutes a popular narrative within the diabetes device industry that positions open source as a practice that exists in opposition to regulators, conjuring the figure of the “rogue” hacker operating in defiance of institutions that exist to promote safety and public health [55]. Yet as this developer explained to me, echoing a belief consistently voiced by Tidepool’s developers, open source is not inherently at odds with regulation. Rather, open source practices, especially when embedded in an organizational culture of "radical transparency," have the potential to bolster the regulation and safety of medical devices [56].

In contrast to the figure of the rogue hacker, none of the Tidepool developers I interviewed (many of whom were also volunteer contributors to DIY projects) were opposed to regulation. Indeed, many of them—almost all of whom had diabetes or were parents to children with diabetes—desired regulated, commercial systems they would not have to build themselves. This was part of what made working for Tidepool attractive. Like its DIY counterparts, Tidepool was developing software that met the software geek's definition of good software. At the same time, as one developer explained, Tidepool was "also something that's easy to sign up for and it's something that's regulated…It's an intersection of all of those needs." The prospect of an FDA-cleared, institutionally supported product that did not compromise on safety was exciting.

The previous sentence might, upon first read, sound nonsensical. FDA clearance, after all, is shorthand for safety, making the promise of a safe FDA-cleared product redundant. But, even within the FDA, "safety" is neither static nor singular; it is a concept with multiple meanings and dimensions whose relative importance is subject to ongoing negotiation. Qualitative studies of DIY Loopers have found, for example, that people using DIY systems carefully weigh different aspects of safety, generally concluding that the improved glycemic outcomes automation confers make conventional therapy the riskier option in comparison, even if the automated system available to them is unregulated ([14], p. 552). What DIY systems lacked in regulation, they made up for in transparency, permitting their users to see the computing logic behind insulin dosing decisions. In this respect, these systems achieved a conception of safety that closed, proprietary systems did not. Take, for instance, this example a developer shared with me about his type 1 daughter's experience using a commercial system:

> It's a magic black box. At some point it started misbehaving and doing weird things. And I was like: I don't know why it's doing this…I've got no way of finding out why it's making these decisions. I can't even tweak any settings. It looked to me like it had the wrong insulin to carb ratio, but it's a black box. I couldn't change it. So I couldn't do anything to improve the results.

When the developer contacted the manufacturer for assistance, the company's representatives were similarly in the dark, unable to explain what precisely had gone awry. "It was a black box. I had no way of figuring out what was going on," he continued. That's when I finally decided to ditch it all together." Concern over commercial systems' opacity, however, is not limited to people with diabetes and software developers. As one endocrinologist explained to me, clinicians, too, lack detailed insight into how the proprietary systems they prescribe make therapy decisions:

> What I really have found unsettling is that so much of what is supposed to be an academic pursuit—of, you know, how do these systems work?— is [instead] all talk about 'we target this number or that number.' That's just a constant…But you're not saying: 'How do I make a dose decision?' …When [companies are] discussing, 'oh hey, we have this great new

> system that achieves 70 percent time in range,' nobody asks: 'Great. How does it work?' That's what I'm interested in knowing and nobody seems to be discussing that... Why is it that this algorithm that has to be intellectual property? What is it that is so special or important about how to deliver insulin—which was supposed to be a free and accessible thing—that you cannot tell people how it works down to the code?

In this physician's comment, two distinct approaches to evidence-generation are apparent, one rooted in clinical research and the other in engineering logics. In medicine, safety and efficacy are evidenced through clinical studies (ideally randomized controlled trials). The focus is on demonstrating the statistical outcomes of an intervention (like a device or a drug) rather than investigating how the intervention works—a task left to "basic science" [57]. Assuming stability between the experimental conditions of the study and everyday life, and the representativeness of the study population, the expectation is that people in the "real world" (i.e., in life outside of the study) will experience largely similar outcomes to those observed in the study population. In software development, in contrast, the key to evaluating a device lies in both understanding how the machine operates and how it performs in the real world. The expectation is continuous change, not stability. "Good" software is made iteratively through regular updates to the software based on user feedback.

Though different, these two expert approaches to evidence are not incompatible. As DiSimone explained to me, "Both are valuable tools for safety. I don't think they exist contrary to each other. I think they both work in tandem." However, without access to the underlying algorithms and source code, a key form of evidence needed to evaluate the device from an engineering perspective is missing. DiSimone added: "I would love to see the commercial side recognize that transparency is better for the patient...I'm sure it's the financial implications that drives [the decision] about releasing that kind of information."

The #wearenotwaiting community is not the only group rethinking what safety means in the era of software-based medical devices. The FDA, too, is engaged in reformulating their review process to better account for the unique properties of software, which pose a challenge to current regulatory frameworks. Since 1976, the FDA has taken a product-by-product strategy for conducting regulatory reviews, meaning that each product is evaluated based on clinical trial data prior to becoming commercially available [58]. In this regulatory framework, the bulk of the review process happens up front during the product's pre-market phase in an effort to predict and prevent potential harm. This framework is based on a set of assumptions about the stability and durability of hardware—namely that the device will stay the same throughout the review process and following commercialization. It assumes that the risk of using a product once it is made commercially available should be about the same as the risk of using the product at the time it was submitted for review. However, in the case of software, the assumption of a relatively stable and unchanging product does not hold up.

Unlike a hardware-based device, which can take years to build and test, software can be built quickly and involves constant iteration and modification—a challenge for regulators sometimes called the "update problem" [59]. "Software moves fast because of iteration...The Facebook mantra—'move fast and break [things]'—you don't want that mantra for a medical device. That would not go well. There is something in the middle," Look explained. Moreover, in modern computing, software almost always spills over the boundaries of a single device, communicating and combining with other devices (including non-medical consumer products like smart phones). As software-based medical devices grow increasingly modifiable and complex (especially with the rapid development of AI/ML), so too do the limitations of current regulations and the challenges facing regulators [5, 58]. The FDA's efforts to respond to these challenges have, according to social studies of regulatory science, led to changes within the FDA itself including a substantial rethinking of regulatory frameworks and an openness to alternative forms of evidence ([60], p. 550). Though popularly scapegoated for "slowing" innovation, in the case of medical software, the FDA has positioned themselves as an "innovation enabler" as much as a "safety watchdog" [60].

Take, for example, the FDA's "Software Precertification (Pre-Cert) Pilot Program," an experiment in regulatory process that involved nine pilot participants, including Tidepool. Likened by FDA officials to the TSA Pre✓® at the airport, which allows travelers who have applied and passed a background check to speed through the security protocols, in the Pre-Cert model organizations undergo an "Excellence Appraisal," essentially the FDA's equivalent to the TSA's background check [61]. After demonstrating "a robust culture of quality and organizational excellence," the pre-certified developer would be allowed to "skip the line" of the normal review process, speeding lower-risk products through FDA clearance and emphasizing post-market surveillance. In a report following the pilot's conclusion, the FDA concluded that the program exceeded the agency's current statutory authorities and required legislative action to be implemented [58]. Nonetheless, the Pre-Cert pilot program illustrates how the problem of software's modifiability is prompting regulators to think about the relationship between software-based medical devices and public health in new ways. Perhaps most notably, the pilot shifted the object of regulation from the product to the process of device development—or, in the pilot program's terms, to the developer's "culture of quality." However, as critics of the program—including Senators Elizabeth Warren (D-Mass), Patty Murray (D-Wash), and Tina Smith (D-Minn)—have pointed out, what precisely constitutes a "culture of quality and organizational excellence" and how it can be evaluated remains a source of ambiguity [62].

Talking with Tidepool's developers, I came to understand Tidepool's cultural commitment to transparency combined with its open source approach to device development as one possible vision for regulation beyond the current regulatory framework.[19] As one developer explained to me, "We're going to be open with everything. I think that's going to make it easier for the FDA to do things because

---

[19] All pilot participants in the Pre-Cert program also underwent the standard review process. Under their cleared Regulatory Quality System, Tidepool will be able to release minor updates to their software (e.g., bug fixes) without seeking regulatory clearance. Substantial updates will require additional review. This approach is consistent with a traditional pre-market (rather than continuous risk-monitoring) framework for medical device regulation [59].

they don't have to worry about giving up company secrets. All of our documents can be online. Anybody can look at them." This transparency extended to Tidepool's code, a type of openness that created (in one developer's words) "the potential for open software to be much safer than proprietary software because you can have outside experts looking at it." Or as another put it, "The more eyeballs there are, the more people look at it, and have the opportunity to perhaps discover something we missed." Open source, in short, created an opportunity for peer review that was not possible when code was shrouded in secrecy.

The developers I spoke with also resoundingly rejected another popular argument against openness. If everything is "out there," what is stopping nefarious actors from hacking personal health data? This narrative, Tidepool developers explained to me, was a gross misconception. "There is a term 'security by obscurity.' If you don't know how a gizmo works, it's secure. That's a complete fallacy," one engineer told me. Another team member offered this analogy: Open source software, they explained, is like "an open-air museum where we invite people to walk in with a lock box in the middle of it." Everyone is invited to see how the museum (i.e., software) works. They know where the lock box (where personal information is stored) is located, but that does not mean they can open it. The lock is designed to be a strong defense. "Almost all encryption protocols that are in use today are published in the open because that gives them a chance to be audited, to be inspected for bugs so that they can be improved," another engineer explained.[20] "Security by obscurity," in contrast, relies on concealing the "museum" altogether in hopes the door remain secret. Indeed, it was this obscurity-based approach that enabled the DIY community to send commands to their insulin pumps in the first place.[21] To be clear, openness alone does not make software secure nor does software have to be open source to be secure. But relying upon secrecy alone is not a reassuring strategy for security.

Though the developers I interviewed believed open source to be a pragmatic solution to many of the challenges facing medical software, they were also adamant that open source is not a panacea. Just as there is variation in proprietary software development, there is variation in open source projects. Assigning software an open source license does not guarantee the software will be good, as this developer explained:

> If you have open software that has nobody outside in the industry looking at it, then it's entirely dependent upon the software process of the company developing. The open isn't actually having any influence on it. And if there's a company developing proprietary soft-

[20] Open source and data privacy are not at odds. Indeed, Tidepool's first value is that "people with diabetes own their data." This value translates into software design that grants users control over where their data goes.

[21] In an interview with the *Prognosis* podcast, Ben West—one of the key contributors to the first DIY AID system, Open APS—drew on a similar metaphor to explain how he initially hacked a Medtronic pump: "It's more like the front door wasn't put on" [63]. Once West found the door, all he had to do was walk right through.

ware with better software processes, better quality assurance processes, they're going to end up with a better product.

The added safety benefits of open source, in other words, were contingent upon other experts taking the time to look. However, peer review is not guaranteed. As the stories of Tidepool and DIY Loop both illustrate, open source projects require a great deal of organizational work to be successful. Still, open source licensing itself does at least create the possibility for external peer review. This same developer continued: "By default, open source is probably going to be the better route because it does give the potential for outside experts to look at it to review it." Loop, he said, was a good example. "We have had a lot of people looking at that code. A lot of people checking in on it, reading it, revising it, updating it and if it was just a small company working on this proprietary wise, we wouldn't have had that nearly that coverage."

Open source creates the opportunity for transparency and collaboration; however, the use of open source, as a pragmatic approach to software development, does not assure an organization's commitment or adherence to either ethic. As open source has transitioned from a controversial legal hack to a commonplace methodology, it has grown further detached from the political and ethical commitments that accompanied its invention [34, 37]. Today, the differences between open source projects can be as important as the differences between open source and proprietary development. Tidepool, for example, modeled itself after Mozilla, the open source community behind the Firefox browser that advocates for an open and accessible internet that respects user's data privacy, drawing on cultural ideals and ethical values reminiscent of free software's origins [64]. Not all organizations who use open source, however, are permeated by the same ethic of transparency and collaboration throughout their operations. Nor are they necessarily committed to the same ethic of data ownership, access, and privacy as Mozilla or Tidepool. Though open source affords the possibility of transparency and collaboration, its use is not necessarily indicative of an organization's wider operating culture or ethical stances.

"It's Not Impossible"

Open source is more than a technical, legal, or economic production model for software development. It is also, according to Christopher Kelty, an anthropologist of free and open source software, a form of argumentation that seeks to persuade not through speech acts, but through "the production of actually existing alternatives" ([21, 65], p. 3). This conception of open source as a form of "argument-by-technology" seems consistent with Tidepool's mission. As Tidepool's Brandon Arbiter, told me, reflecting upon the organization's decision to make its software open source, "We wanted to be open source so that we can help spur innovation—so that we can show the device companies how to do it. We can show them that it's not impossible." By using open source software, Tidepool's aim was not just to create the specific technology they wanted to see exist, though that was certainly part of it. Their goal was and remains fundamentally reformist: to improve the diabetes device industry by proving to the big companies that the interoperable devices they desire—as both software developers and people living with diabetes—are not far-fetched visions for the future but practical and feasible solutions in the present.

It is far from guaranteed that Tidepool Loop, as both a product and argument, will find success or, for that matter, that open source will follow a similar trajectory in health care as in other industries. As the history of science and technology teaches us, the evolution of technology is highly contingent, not preordained [66, 67]. In an industry where proprietary software remains the default approach, open source may create new possibilities for software development and regulation, but how it will materialize in health care depends very much on the actors involved and the broader political-economic milieu in which it is embedded. "Medtronic could decide to be an open source company like Microsoft decided to be an open source company. They're not entirely open source but they have huge swaths of the company that are open source. Any traditional medical device company could decide to be open source. None of them have, but they could," Look explained during our interview.

Tidepool Loop's story also complicates narratives that figure regulators solely as innovation barriers. To be sure, Tidepool team members, like the FDA itself, believe there is a mismatch between current regulatory models and modern software development—a mismatch the FDA's (now concluded) Pre-Cert pilot program set out to address. In other cases, the FDA has actually paved the way for new approaches to diabetes software. Tidepool Loop's clearance, for example, materializes the pathway the FDA outlined for third-party interoperability. However, for Tidepool Loop to actually be commercially released, and to make the full vision of "mixing and matching" AID system components a reality, other device manufacturers will need to pursue this regulatory clearance too—and "no authority exists to enforce cooperation" ([54, 68], p. 61). Though several commercially available pumps have achieved the ACE pump designation, at the time of writing in 2023, no pump manufacturer had yet sought the third-party control (i.e., clearance to work with software and algorithms other than their own proprietary systems) [4]. As Tidepool Loop's clearance evidences, it is not the FDA that is preventing this reality.

In recent years, there has been a growing movement to value and incorporate user feedback and patient experience data into the medical device development and evaluation process.[22] This is an important development in the making of medical devices. However, insights from this case study suggest that listening to user feedback (as important as it is) may do little to change how medical software operates if the conditions for developers to act on that feedback are not in place. In this sense, this chapter serves as an invitation to also listen to the people making medical software—not to the hype of consumer technology companies but to the practical realities of individuals responsible for developing the technologies users desire and

[22] The incorporation of the INSPIRE measure in the evaluation of AID systems is an important example of the movement toward valuing patient experiences [69].

expect. These practical realities—and the value judgments and political-economic conditions that underlie them—have consequences for what the technologies patients and clinicians rely upon can do. To be clear, open source will not fix all the challenges facing medical software. The adoption of industry standards, for example, remains a critical step [70]. There is also no guarantee that, in the absence of larger social transformation and health system reform, products developed using open source will be distributed more equitably than their proprietary counterparts [71, 72]. And though transparency can help, open source is not the only solution required to ensure trustworthy and accountable technology amidst rapid developments in AI/ML [5, 73]. But open source *is* a solution to a particular problem that software developers *and* regulators face—a problem that may only increase in import as the digitization of health care continues to unfold.

Acknowledgments Research for this chapter was supported by a National Science Foundation Graduate Research Fellowship. I want to thank Hatice Nilay Erten, Kathryn Goldfarb, Jordan Herman, Christopher Snider, and Jennifer Wagner for their generous engagement with various iterations of this chapter. My sincerest gratitude to Christopher Snider and the Tidepool team for welcoming this project and my questions, and to all my interlocutors for their thoughtful contributions.

The DIY Loop community lost one of its most dedicated contributors and leaders when Katie DiSimone passed away from glioblastoma in 2023 [73]. The outpouring of support and gratitude from the Looper community throughout Katie's cancer journey and following her passing testify to the difference she made in the lives of thousands of people with diabetes and their families. Thank you, Katie.

References

1. Briskin A. Tidepool expands closed loop access. Wins Clearance From FDA. diaTribe; 2023.
2. Park A. Tidepool lands long-awaited FDA nod for diabetes management app. Fierce Biotech; 2023.
3. Lee M. Interoperability is the how, not the why. Tidepool Blog; 2020. https://www.tidepool.org/blog/interoperability-is-the-how-not-the-why. Accessed 5 Feb 2023.
4. Look H. Third party control for ACE pumps. Tidepool Blog; 2023. https://www.tidepool.org/blog/the-inside-scoop-on-third-party-control-for-ace-pumps. Accessed 16 Feb 2023.
5. Gerke S, Babic B, Evgeniou T, Cohen IG. The need for a system view to regulate artificial intelligence/machine learning-based software as medical device. NPJ Digit Med. 2020;3:53. https://doi.org/10.1038/s41746-020-0262-2.
6. Gardler R, Walli S. Evolving perspective on community and governance. In: Brock A, editor. Open source law, policy and practice. 2nd ed. Oxford University Press; 2022. p. 34–67.
7. OSI. The open source definition. Open Source Initiative; 2007. https://opensource.org/docs/osd.
8. Walden I. Open source as philosophy, methodology, and commerce: using law with attitude. In: Brock A, editor. Open source law, policy and practice. 2nd ed. Oxford University Press; 2022. p. 1–33.
9. Burnside MJ, Lewis DM, Crocket HR, et al. Open-source automated insulin delivery in type 1 diabetes. N Engl J Med. 2022;387:869–81. https://doi.org/10.1056/NEJMoa2203913.

10. Lewis D. Understanding the difference between open source and DIY in diabetes. DIYPS.org; 2022. https://diyps.org/2022/09/28/understanding-the-difference-between-open-source-and-diy-in-diabetes/. Accessed 22 Dec 2022.
11. Crabtree TS, McLay A, Wilmot EG. DIY artificial pancreas systems: here to stay? Pract Diabetes. 2019;36:63–8. https://doi.org/10.1002/pdi.2216.
12. Dinneen SF, McMorrow L. Re-framing type 1 diabetes care through open-source automated insulin delivery: 'The (expert) patient will see you now, doctor'. Diabetes Med. 2022;39:e14839. https://doi.org/10.1111/dme.14839.
13. Lum JW, Bailey RJ, Barnes-Lomen V, et al. A real-world prospective study of the safety and effectiveness of the loop open source automated insulin delivery system. Diabetes Technol Ther. 2021;23:367–75. https://doi.org/10.1089/dia.2020.0535.
14. Schipp J, Skinner T, Holloway E, et al. How adults with type 1 diabetes are navigating the challenges of open-source artificial pancreas systems: a qualitative study. Diabetes Technol Ther. 2021;23:546–54. https://doi.org/10.1089/dia.2020.0652.
15. Schipp J, Skinner TC, Holloway E, et al. 'We're all on the same team'. Perspectives on the future of artificial pancreas systems by adults in Australia with type 1 diabetes using open-source technologies: a qualitative study. Diabetes Med. 2022;39:e14708. https://doi.org/10.1111/dme.14708.
16. Suttiratana SC, Wong JJ, Lanning MS, et al. Qualitative study of user experiences with loop, an open-source automated insulin delivery system. Diabetes Technol Ther. 2022;24:416–23. https://doi.org/10.1089/dia.2021.0485.
17. Wolf AS. OPEN—Launch—The OPEN Project. 2019. https://open-diabetes.eu/en/open-launch/. Accessed 20 Dec 2022.
18. Gottlieb SD. The fantastical empowered patient. In: Healthcare activism. Oxford University Press; 2021. p. 198–223.
19. Jansky B, Langstrup H. Device activism and material participation in healthcare: retracing forms of engagement in the #WeAreNotWaiting movement for open-source closed-loop systems in type 1 diabetes self-care. BioSocieties. 2022;18:498. https://doi.org/10.1057/s41292-022-00278-4.
20. Goldstein DM, Hall K. Mass hysteria in Le Roy, New York: how brain experts materialized truth and outscienced environmental inquiry: how brain experts materialized truth. Am Ethnol. 2015;42:640–57. https://doi.org/10.1111/amet.12161.
21. Kelty C. Two bits: the cultural significance of free software. Duke University Press; 2008.
22. DiabetesMine. The #WeAreNotWaiting DIY diabetes movement. Healthline; 2019.
23. Sabicer S. Tandem diabetes care launches first ever remote software update for insulin pump using a personal computer. 2017.
24. Kennedy L, Brown A. FDA approves Dexcom G5 CGM for insulin dosing. diaTribe; 2016.
25. Talking About Tidepool Loop and Telemedicine with Howard Look. CWDiabetes; 2020.
26. Look H. #WeAreNotWaiting. the (not so?) brief story of Tidepool. Six until me diabetes blog. In: Six until me. 2015. https://sixuntilme.com/wp/2015/01/19/wearenotwaiting-brief-story-tidepool/. Accessed 2 Apr 2021.
27. Whitney E. Datapalooza: a concept, a conference and a movement. NPR; 2013.
28. Schulte F, Fortune EF. Death by 1,000 clicks: where electronic health records went wrong. Kaiser Health News. 2019; https://khn.org/news/death-by-a-thousand-clicks/. Accessed 10 Oct 2022.
29. Mandl KD, Kohane IS. Data standards may be wonky, but they will transform health care—STAT. Stat News. 2019.
30. Rivera L. What SMART on FHIR means for the future of healthcare. auth0 blog. 2021.
31. Picton PE, Yeung M, Hamming N, et al. Advancement of the artificial pancreas through the development of interoperability standards. J Diabetes Sci Technol. 2013;7:1066–70. https://doi.org/10.1177/193229681300700431.
32. OSI. Open standards requirement for software. Open Source Initiative; 2006. https://opensource.org/osr. Accessed 5 Feb 2023.

33. Siegel J, Soley RM. Open source and open standards: working together for effective software development and distribution. Open Source Business Resource; 2008.
34. Coleman G. CODE IS SPEECH: legal tinkering, expertise, and protest among free and open source software developers. Cult Anthropol. 2009;24:420–54. https://doi.org/10.1111/j.1548-1360.2009.01036.x.
35. Hernandez D. Tech time warp of the week: watch Steve Ballmer Mock Linux while dressed as the Matrix's neo. Wired. 2014.
36. Stallman R. Why open source misses the point of free software—GNU project—Free Software Foundation. GNU Operating System. n.d. https://www.gnu.org/philosophy/open-source-misses-the-point.en.html. Accessed 2 Dec 2022.
37. Kelty C. There is no free software. J Peer Product. 2013;1:3.
38. Metz C. Meet Bill Gates, the man who changed open source software. Wired. 2012.
39. Microsoft. Microsoft to acquire GitHub for $7.5 billion. Stories. 2018. https://news.microsoft.com/2018/06/04/microsoft-to-acquire-github-for-7-5-billion/. Accessed 31 Mar 2023.
40. Sundar N. Forks and branches. NITRR Open Source; 2020. https://medium.com/nitrr-open-source/forks-and-branches-git-ninja-83980a370080. Accessed 5 Feb 2023.
41. Look H. Tidepool original strategy document: a a disruptive, open approach to diabetes care. 2013.
42. León-Vargas F, Martin C, Garcia-Jaramillo M, et al. Is a cloud-based platform useful for diabetes management in Colombia? The Tidepool experience. Comput Methods Prog Biomed. 2021;208:106205. https://doi.org/10.1016/j.cmpb.2021.106205.
43. Selmer C, Green A, Johannesen M, et al. Stenopool: a system for managing all diabetes device data. Diabetes Technology & Therapeutics. Mary Ann/Liebert, Inc. Publishers, p OP041 #220; 2022.
44. Nafus, Neff G. Self-tracking. MIT Press; 2016.
45. Kaziunas E, Ackerman MS, Lindtner S, Lee JM. Caring through data: attending to the social and emotional experiences of health datafication. In: Proceedings of the 2017 ACM Conference on Computer Supported Cooperative Work and Social Computing—CSCW '17. Portland, Oregon: ACM Press; 2017. p. 2260–72.
46. Kaziunas E, Lindtner S, Ackerman MS, Lee JM. Lived data: tinkering with bodies, code, and care work. Human Comput Interact. 2018;33:49–92. https://doi.org/10.1080/07370024.2017.1307749.
47. Lewis D. History and perspective on DIY closed looping. J Diabetes Sci Technol. 2019;13:790–3. https://doi.org/10.1177/1932296818808307.
48. Racklyeft N. The history of Loop and LoopKit. Medium. 2016. https://medium.com/@loudnate/the-history-of-loop-and-loopkit-59b3caf13805. Accessed 1 Feb 2021.
49. Gardler R, Hanganu G. Benevolent dictator governance model. OSS Watch; 2010.
50. Tidepool. In memory of Katie DiSimone. Tidepool. 2023. https://www.tidepool.org/katie-disimone. Accessed 31 Mar 2023.
51. OpenAPS. Frequently asked questions—OpenAPS.org. OPENAPS.ORG. n.d. https://openaps.org/frequently-asked-questions/. Accessed 5 Feb 2023.
52. Loop. Welcome to loop. LoopDocs. n.d. https://loopkit.github.io/loopdocs/. Accessed 5 Feb 2023.
53. Herrick B. AID systems compatibility and interoperability workshop. JDRF; 2018. https://www.jdrf.org/blog/2018/03/23/aid-systems-compatibility-interoperability-workshop/. Accessed 5 Feb 2023.
54. Parmar A. When it comes to diabetes devices and apps, FDA prefers mixing and matching—MedCity News. MedCity News; 2019.
55. Gottlieb SD, Cluck J. Going rogue. Digit Cult Soc. 2018;4:137–56. https://doi.org/10.14361/dcs-2018-0208.
56. Snider C. How radical transparency is transforming open source healthcare software. Opensource.com. 2022. https://opensource.com/article/22/2/transparency-open-source-healthcare-software. Accessed 5 Feb 2023.

57. Timmermans S, Berg M. The gold standard: the challenge of evidence-based medicine and standardization in health care. Temple University Press; 2003.
58. FDA. FDA regulation of mobile medical apps. FDA; 2022.
59. Babic B, Gerke S, Evgeniou T, Cohen IG. Algorithms on regulatory lockdown in medicine. Science. 2019;366:1202–4. https://doi.org/10.1126/science.aay9547.
60. Lievevrouw E, Marelli L, Van Hoyweghen I. The FDA's standard-making process for medical digital health technologies: co-producing technological and organizational innovation. BioSocieties. 2022;17:549–76. https://doi.org/10.1057/s41292-021-00232-w.
61. Evans B. Podcast: the current state of digital health regulation. Rock Health. 2019.
62. Lovett L. Trio of US senators continue to question FDA's PreCert efforts. MobiHealthNews; 2019.
63. Kresge N, Cortez MF. The $250 Biohack that's revolutionizing life with diabetes. 2018. Bloomberg.com.
64. Mozilla. Who we are. Mozilla Foundation; 2019. https://foundation.mozilla.org/en/who-we-are/. Accessed 5 Feb 2023.
65. Kelty C. Geeks, social imaginaries, and recursive publics. Cult Anthropol. 2005;20:185–214. https://doi.org/10.1525/can.2005.20.2.185.
66. Epstein S. Impure science: AIDS, activism, and the politics of knowledge. University of California Press; 1998.
67. Latour B. Science in action: how to follow scientists and engineers through society. Harvard University Press; 1988.
68. Braune K, Lal RA, Petruželková L, et al. Open-source automated insulin delivery: international consensus statement and practical guidance for health-care professionals. Lancet Diabetes Endocrinol. 2022;10:58–74. https://doi.org/10.1016/S2213-8587(21)00267-9.
69. Weissberg-Benchell J, Shapiro JB, Hood K, et al. Assessing patient-reported outcomes for automated insulin delivery systems: the psychometric properties of the INSPIRE measures. Diabetes Med. 2019;36:644–52. https://doi.org/10.1111/dme.13930.
70. Espinoza J, Klonoff DC, Vidmar A, et al. Integration of continuous glucose monitor data into the electronic health record. Diabetes Technology Society; 2022.
71. Dunbar-Hester C. Hacking diversity: the politics of inclusion in open technology cultures. Princeton, NJ: Princeton University Press; 2020.
72. Hatch AR, Gordon JT, Sternlieb SR. The artificial pancreas in cyborg bodies. In: Boero N, Mason K, editors. The Oxford handbook of the sociology of body and embodiment. Oxford University Press; 2020. p. 412–30.
73. Surman M. Introducing Mozilla.ai: investing in trustworthy AI. The Mozilla Blog. dist://ed. 2023. https://blog.mozilla.org/en/mozilla/introducing-mozilla-ai-investing-in-trustworthy-ai/. Accessed 5 Apr 2023.

Index

S. Fishman (ed.), *Advances in Diabetes Technology*, Contemporary Endocrinology, https://doi.org/10.1007/978-3-031-75352-7

D

GPSR Compliance

The European Union's (EU) General Product Safety Regulation (GPSR) is a set of rules that requires consumer products to be safe and our obligations to ensure this.

If you have any concerns about our products, you can contact us on ProductSafety@springernature.com

In case Publisher is established outside the EU, the EU authorized representative is:

Springer Nature Customer Service Center GmbH
Europaplatz 3
69115 Heidelberg, Germany

Batch number: 10726135

Printed by Printforce, the Netherlands